Medicine Free
How Food IS Your Medicine

Bob Avery MD, FACP

Copyright © 2012 Bob Avery MD, FACP

All rights reserved.

ISBN:148127807X
ISBN-13:9781481278072

DEDICATION

I dedicate this book to all my patients past, present and future. Their courage has been absolutely inspirational. I must also thank my family. Without their support and love, I would not have found the time and motivation to write this book. I especially thank my oldest son Bill who was inspired me to finally write a book after he published his first novel.

CONTENTS

	ACKNOWLEDGEMENTS	i
	INTRODUCTION	9
1	WHAT IS HEALTH?	11
2	NUTRIGENOMICS-Natural Healing	43
3	HOW TO TAKE CHARGE OF YOUR HEALTH THROUGH DIET	81
4	PUTTING IT ALL TOGETHER	111
5	MY THOUGHTS ON WHAT MAKES A HEALTHFUL DIET	149
	REFERENCES	179

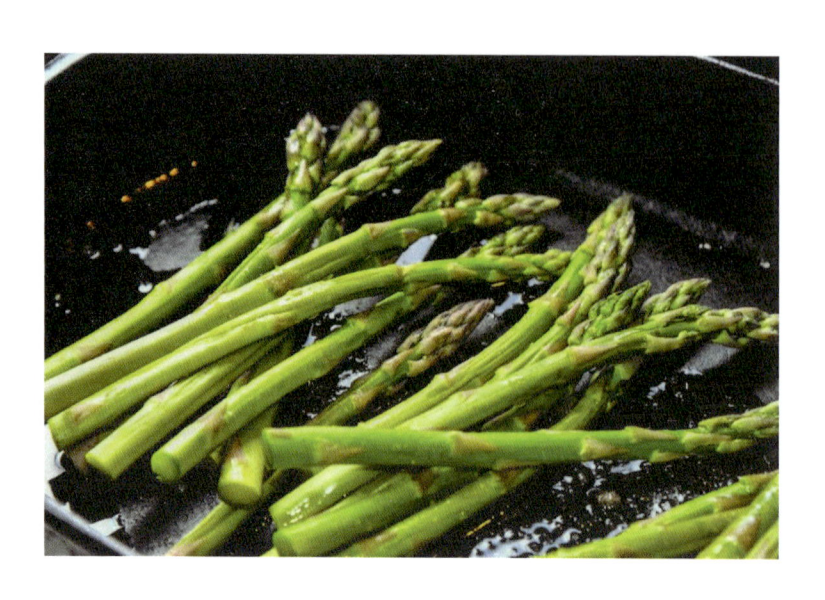

ACKNOWLEDGMENTS

I thank Dr. Taormina Low Dog, Shari Rossmann, and Dominica Avery for reviewing the manuscript, Dr. Randy Jirtle for use of the Agouti mouse photos, Emily Flowers for editing, Margaret Dauber for her artistic input and most of all my wife, Carole, who put up with me during the whole process of writing, editing and publishing, "I'll be home for dinner honey!"

A special thanks to Mark Dauber for his excellent photography. He can be contacted at Daubergallery.com

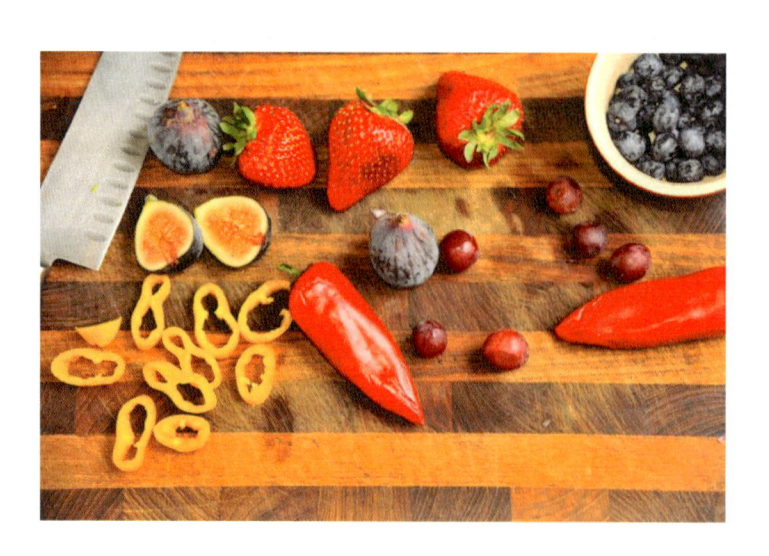

INTRODUCTION

MEDICINE FREE, AT LAST!

Food IS your medicine. How eating certain healthy foods can reverse disease and break your dependence on medicines.

Are you healthy? Do you take blood pressure medicine, diabetes medicine, and heart medicine? You may take a vitamin tablet to be healthy but you are still dependent on medicines. You will also find medicines do not cure high blood pressure, diabetes, or heart disease, they just control the signs of the disease. Finally, do you feel like you are just spending money, making insurance companies and pharmaceutical companies richer, while you don't feel much better? According to the National Center for Health Care Statistics, we spend nearly $7000 per person for health care in this country, and nearly $1700 of that comes out of your pocket! The average person over 65 takes 12 different medicines and the co-pay for them can be as much as $100 each. We pay more than any other country in the world for healthcare and yet we are not healthy. Americans don't even live the longest, we rank 49th in the world in life expectancy. According to the National Center for Healthcare Statistics, 50 million Americans are disabled and 51% of those over the age of 65 have at least mild disability. Do you think we are healthy now? After reading this book, you will understand why vitamins really don't make you healthier and medicines only mask the real problems in our health. There is a way to prevent, reverse, and cure diseases but it isn't sold at the pharmacy. The secret to good health is not in a synthetic vitamin or medicine. The secret to good health is at the grocery store and in your pantry. Your body has amazing mechanisms to become and stay healthy. All you have to do is feed yourself correctly and that is not hard to do once you know some basic rules that I'll explain in this book.

Your mother always said, "Eat your vegetables." She was right. "Eat your vegetables" is one way to stay healthy, but did you ever ask yourself why? Why are they so important? What do they actually do to the body? Up until recently, we could merely suspect that certain foods were associated with good health. New research has unlocked the secrets behind healthy foods and how they change your body. Certain foods and nutrition actually affect you deep in your cells at the DNA level. This is where diseases start and this is where they can be stopped or reversed.

Together, we will explore which foods and nutrients are healthful and why they impact your body's lifelong well-being. Then, working from recent scientific studies in the fields of nutrition, cancer and genetics, we will look at what nutrients in the vegetables are good for you and how nutrients interact with the body. Even if this kind of eating and body maintenance is totally new to you, you will be on your way to avoiding medicines, saving money and achieving better health if you follow these simple recommendations.

1. WHAT IS HEALTH?

I've never been as excited to be a part of medicine as I am now. I've practiced medicine and oncology for over 20 years. Not only do I get to work with truly wonderful and courageous people as I help them through the treatment of the devastating disease, cancer, but the exciting scientific discoveries in medicine are astonishing and occur more frequently now than ever before in history. Medical breakthroughs which were made once a century prior to the 19th century now occur on an annual basis. Never before have we had so much knowledge on how to prevent and treat diseases.

Although the death rate for cancer has dropped steadily over the last 15 years, we have a long way to go to find a cure for all cancers. Heart disease kills nearly 600,000 Americans every year. It is clear cancer and other diseases are extremely difficult to cure once they develop- that's often too late. I'm interested in preventing disease. It is much easier, it is possible, and it is the key to a long and healthy life.

HEALTH AND LIFESTYLE

Lifestyle choices play a major role in the diseases humans face, as research shows again and again. Fighting a patient's lifestyle choices can be frustrating for a physician who can only do so much at a checkup to influence a patient. We can't take the steps of prevention for our patients. It is my hope that after reading this book, you will be empowered to take charge of your life, make changes to your diet and become healthier in a lasting way.

It is common knowledge that certain foods like vegetables, fruit, fish, chicken and lean meat are good for you and we have scientific data to prove it. We also know processed foods, saturated fats, trans-fats, corn oil, fried foods, processed meats and fatty corn fed beef are unhealthy. Did you ever wonder why, exactly, these things have a bad effect on our health? We know bad foods cause oxidation and inflammation, which damage your cells. It is possible to measure damaged protein or DNA that result from oxidation and inflammation, but these foods also affect your health in a more profound way, one that can be passed to your children.

All foods, good or bad, have an effect on your genes. What is a gene? Genes are part of your DNA and they are the blueprint for all the things your cells do. Only a fraction of all your genes are active at any given time; most are turned off. The process of turning genes off and on is called epigenetics. Substances in foods also turn your genes off and on. The study of how food affects your genes is called nutrigenomics. It is a fascinating process that is the focus of a rapidly growing research area.[1] We are now unlocking the processes by which

---

[1] In each of our cells lies a nucleus containing 46 chromosomes. Each chromosome is composed of Deoxyribonucleic acid or DNA. The DNA is composed of genes. The genes are the blueprint of the cell telling it what to do and what to become. Through the human genome project we have identified all the genes in the human body but that did not answer all our questions about health and disease. We only use a fraction of the 20,000 genes in our bodies. Why we have so many extra genes is a mystery. Furthermore, we have discovered that we all have genes that can cause disease in our bodies. That

genes are turned on and off. The study of how genes are turned on and off will open a new world to us. It will help us determine which foods to eat, but also help us develop new medicines to fight disease. These certainly are exciting times – it's possible to learn how to transform your life and your health through better gene management.

THE DEFINITION OF HEALTH

When asked about their health, people usually respond by describing whether or not they are experiencing any symptoms at the moment. If a patient tells their doctor, "I feel healthy," that patient is describing his health as the absence of symptoms. "I don't feel sick, I don't have any aches or pains, so I must be healthy!" This isn't exactly the full story, though. Even if you don't feel sick, sore, or see any obvious symptoms, there can be a serious latent illness present. For example, a man with high blood pressure or high blood cholesterol will not feel sick until he actually has a heart attack or stroke, not aware that the disease has been present for years. Many people are not truly as healthy as they think they are, even though they feel fine. Similarly, there can be a bad gene present in your DNA that will ultimately lead to a major illness, but

---

means we are all at risk of getting very sick unless the bad genes are turned off. Likewise, we have good genes that prevent diseases. When these are turned on, we are healthy. Epigenetics is the study of how genes are turned off and on. Nutrigenomics is the study of how nutrients in the foods we eat can turn on or off genes.

remains hidden until the illness occurs. We know from cancer studies that it can take years for a cell to develop from a normal cell to a widespread cancer. Heart disease, which doesn't lead to problems until adulthood, actually begins in early childhood. The early stages of plaque development can be seen in arteries in children as young as 6 years old. Cold and flu symptoms occur predominantly in the winter months, but the lack of flu symptoms in the summer does not mean we are well. The immune systems functions all year long to prevent infections and remove unwanted cells, including cancer cells. Many people who feel perfectly well are unaware that there may be serious trouble brewing. Absence of symptoms does not mean you are healthy; don't fall into this trap.

What is true health, then? A state of health means all the body processes-the immune system, stem cells, the DNA repair system, regulatory systems, and the major organs like the heart, lungs and blood vessels-are all functioning at their normal level. The difficulty is that these processes aren't visible until a problem occurs, so it is common medical practice for doctors to treat the signs of disease, like high blood pressure or blood sugar, without addressing the root causes of high blood pressure or blood sugar in the first place. That's just controlling problems, not curing them or preventing them. If a patient stops taking blood pressure medicine, his blood pressure will return to dangerous levels. The medicine doesn't fix the fundamental problem. It would be much better to reverse it or better yet, prevent the high blood pressure in the first place. We owe it to ourselves to know how to keep our bodily processes working properly. True health is the goal, true health is a possibility, and true health is dependent on our genes. What we eat directly affects our genes. Do you see the connection now? Diseases can be reversed or prevented by what we eat. That is why it is so important to continue reading.

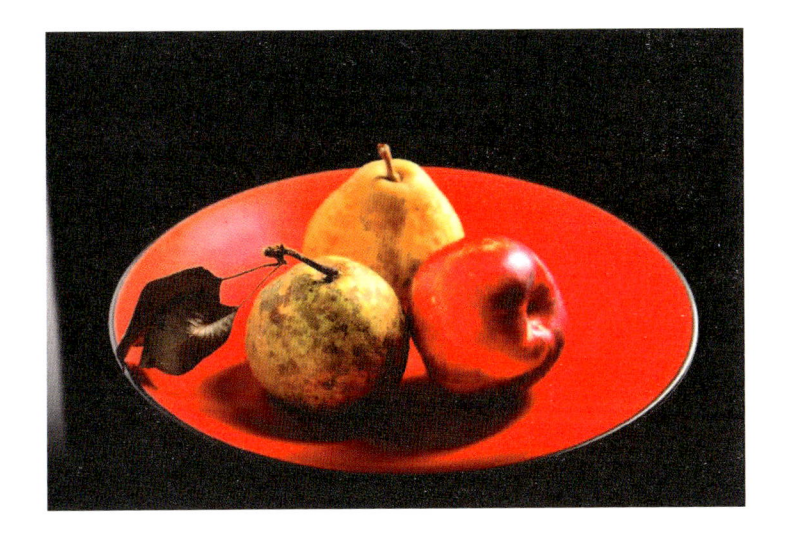

GENES AND EPIGENETICS: HOW DO WE BECOME SICK?[2]

Which diseases are caused by genes?

Genetic diseases occur in a variety of ways.[3] There are genes identified that cause cancers, heart disease, high cholesterol, high blood pressure, Alzheimer's disease, and kidney diseases. In fact most diseases now have an abnormal gene associated with it. Some diseases occur after a gene is mutated or damaged, or sometimes a gene is lost completely. A mutation in a gene can either delete a beneficial gene or

---

[2] What are DNA and genes and how do they work? The discovery of deoxyribonucleic acid (DNA) by Watson and Crick in 1953 changed our knowledge of disease. Watson and Crick were later awarded the Nobel Prize in Medicine in 1964 for their discovery. DNA forms each of the 46 chromosomes in our cells. The DNA is a twisted strand of amino acids. These amino acids are organized into genes and sections to support the genes. The genes are like a blueprint for the cell and they have many functions. They tell a cell what to become, such as a muscle cell or skin cell. They can also set up the mechanism to produce proteins which are the building block for every process in the body. Proteins form cells, cell membranes, blood vessels, muscles, enzymes, hormones, growth factors, and the machinery by which cells grow. Genes are responsible for all these processes but also for health and disease.

[3] There are two copies of genes in our bodies, one from our mother and one from our father. There are many diseases that are inherited from our parents. There are a variety of genetic diseases that affect a variety of organ systems such as sickle cell anemia, cystic fibrosis, polycystic kidney disease, Duchenne muscular dystrophy and hemophilia. In other cases, loss of chromosomes or additional chromosomes are present leading to disease. This is the case in Down's syndrome in which there are 3 copies of the 21st chromosome instead of the normal 2 copies.

can take a normal gene and alter its function. Many colon cancers occur because the genes responsible for repair of damaged DNA are mutated. Another mechanism for cancer occurs when a tumor-causing gene (oncogene) is mutated and turned on. Even so, mutations in genes only lead to a small proportion of diseases. Most diseases are not caused by mutations. They develop when good genes turn off and bad genes turn on. The process of turning genes off or on is directly affected by factors outside of our bodies. Environmental and lifestyle factors- that is, what you eat, drink or smoke - play a major role in how genes behave. What you eat can help good genes work. However, if you don't eat right, bad genes can be turned on causing a variety of diseases. This process of genes getting turned off or on is called epigenetics. How genes are turned on and off not only affects your own health, but the health of your children; these changes can be passed down through three generations. This fact makes it even more important than previously believed to eat healthful food and live a healthy life. You are affecting the health of your children and grandchildren as well.

GENEVITABILITY

If you have an abnormal gene you should get the disease associated with that gene. That is what many people think. This makes diseases not just inevitable but also *gene*vitable. New technologies enable us to rapidly and easily analyze tissues for the genes that are expressed. This research has discovered many new genes that are associated with a variety of diseases. We have identified genes that lead to Alzheimer's disease, heart disease, cancers, high blood pressure, depression and many others. The evening news seems to report on a new gene every few months. In one way this is exciting, but in another it can be depressing. The study of genes and disease would leave you to think there is no control over our health. Taking away control only makes us stressed and depressed, but I am here to give you back your control.

There is no inevitable link between having certain genes and developing the related disease. Nowhere has this been demonstrated so conclusively as in the following study. A group of normal volunteers without illnesses or evidence of blood diseases was tested for the presence of the gene that causes chronic myeloid leukemia.[4] The researchers found that 1 out of every 3 of the study subjects had the gene that causes chronic myeloid leukemia. This would suggest that 30% of the population or 100,000,000 Americans will get chronic myeloid leukemia sometime in their life. The actual risk is much lower, only 1 in 100,000. That means that of the 100 million Americans with the abnormal gene, only 1,000 will get the disease. Those are pretty good odds. This case highlights the point that having a gene does not mean you will get the disease. There are other factors involved. This is

---

[4] Chronic myeloid leukemia occurs when a portion of the 9th chromosome translocates or moves to the 22nd chromosome. This translocation, written as t(9;22), is called the Philadelphia chromosome. The translocation moves the Abelson cancer gene (abl) on chromosome 9 to the Breakpoint Cluster Region (bcr) on chromosome 22 (bcr-abl). This translocation directly leads to the disease.

where epigenetics comes in.

EPIGENETICS

Epigenetic explains how we can have bad genes but never get their associated diseases. There are several ways in which genes are controlled in the cell. One way is to hide the gene. When the DNA is wrapped tightly in the cell, genes on the inside of the coil are not exposed and cannot be turned off or on. The DNA in your cells is very long. In fact, the DNA in each cell is about 1 ½ inches long and it must fit into a cell that is 1/10,000 of an inch in size. To fit in the cell the DNA is wound tightly around a spool.[5] This not only makes the DNA fit into the

---

[5] There are 46 chromosomes in every cell of your body. The DNA in each chromosome is very long. In fact, if you unwound one chromosome, the DNA would be 1 ½ inches long. The chromosomes from one whole cell would be 6 feet long and if you placed all the chromosomes from your whole body end to end, the strand would be long enough to reach the sun and back 70 times! That is an incredible amount of DNA to put in a typical human cell which is 4/10,000 of an inch in diameter. To fit in the cell, the DNA is tightly coiled around a spool called a histone. You can imagine that when the DNA is tightly coiled up the genes would be hidden from view and would not be activated. The chemical process that opens or closes the histone coil is called acetylation. An acetyl group is shown in the figure here.

Acetyl Group

It is composed of 2 carbons, 3 hydrogens, and 1 oxygen. When the acetyl group is attached to the histone, it changes the electrical charge of the histone, which loosens its grip on the DNA. As the DNA unwinds, genes are exposed and can be acted upon to produce proteins. When the acetyl groups are removed, the

cell but it also helps protect the DNA. When the cell needs to divide a chemical reaction unwinds the DNA off the spool and allows the genes to be acted upon. Another way a gene is controlled is through a chemical on/off switch. This is present at the beginning of every gene. When a chemical group called a methyl group attaches to the gene, it turns it off. Remove the methyl group and the gene turns on. This sounds complex and not related to your diet, but here is the interesting part. We now know that certain healthy foods actually change the expression of genes by these various chemical processes. What you eat does matter, because of its effect on turning on good genes and turning off bad genes. Biochemistry and food are linked and it is the most important association for your health.

---

electrical charge changes again and the histone tightens. The enzymes responsible for this are called acetylases because they place acetyl groups on the histone. There are also enzymes that remove them called de-acetylases. This is one form of a chemical on/off switch. When you acetylate the histone, the DNA unwinds and gene activation occurs. When you remove the acetyl group, the DNA binds tight to the histone and genes are turned off.

$$H_3C-\xi$$
Methyl Group

Another form of gene regulation is an on/off switch at the site of the gene. There is an on/off switch before each gene called a promoter region. When the promoter is activated, it promotes or turns on the gene. This also has a chemical on/off switch called the methyl group. When the methyl groups are attached to the promoter site, the gene is turned off. So even if it is exposed by the histone, it will not be activated. When the methyl groups are removed, the gene turns on and starts working. The enzymes responsible for placing the methyl groups are called methyl-transferases because they transfer methyl groups to the promoter region. There are other processes involved in gene activation, but these are the two main mechanisms to turn genes on and off and we will find out later how food nutrients has effects on histones and promoter methylation.

EXAMPLES OF EPIGENETICS IN COMMON DISEASES

There are thousands of studies of epigenetics and its role in the function of cells. Since we are interested in the studies on health, let's look at some examples of how epigenetics plays a role in common diseases such as obesity, metabolic syndrome, diabetes, heart disease and cancer.

Obesity has become an epidemic in the United States and the world.[6] According to the Centers for Disease Control and Prevention (CDC) 33.8% or about 1/3 of adults and 17% of children and adolescents are obese. There has been a dramatic increase in obesity rates over the last 20 years. In 1990, of the states participating in the Behavior Risk Factor Surveillance System, 10 states had an obesity rate of less than 10% and no state had a rate higher than 15%. By 2000, no state had an obesity rate of less than 10% and 23 states had a rate of up to 25%. In 2010, no state had an obesity rate of less than 20%, and 12 states had an obesity

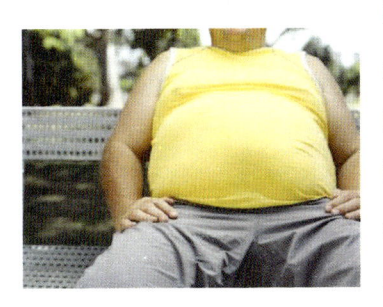

---

[6] Obesity is determined by your height and weight and is measured as body mass index (BMI). A BMI of > 25kg/m2 is considered overweight, a BMI of > 30 kg/m2 is considered obese. Calculators to determine your BSA are available on the internet, or you can use this table from the National Institutes of Health. A table from the National Institutes of Health appears on page 24.

rate of equal to or greater than 30%. See the picture on the next page. The following page contains a chart that will help you determine if you are overweight or obese. Obesity is a national crisis that has scientists and politicians scrambling for answers and treatments.

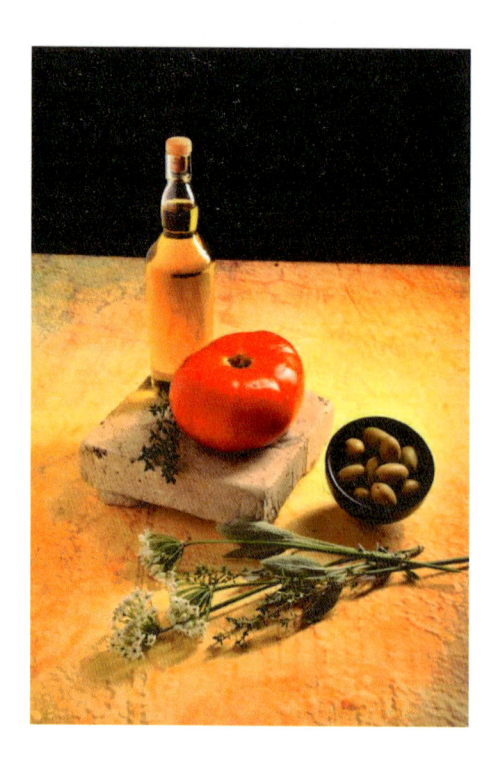

MEDICINE FREE

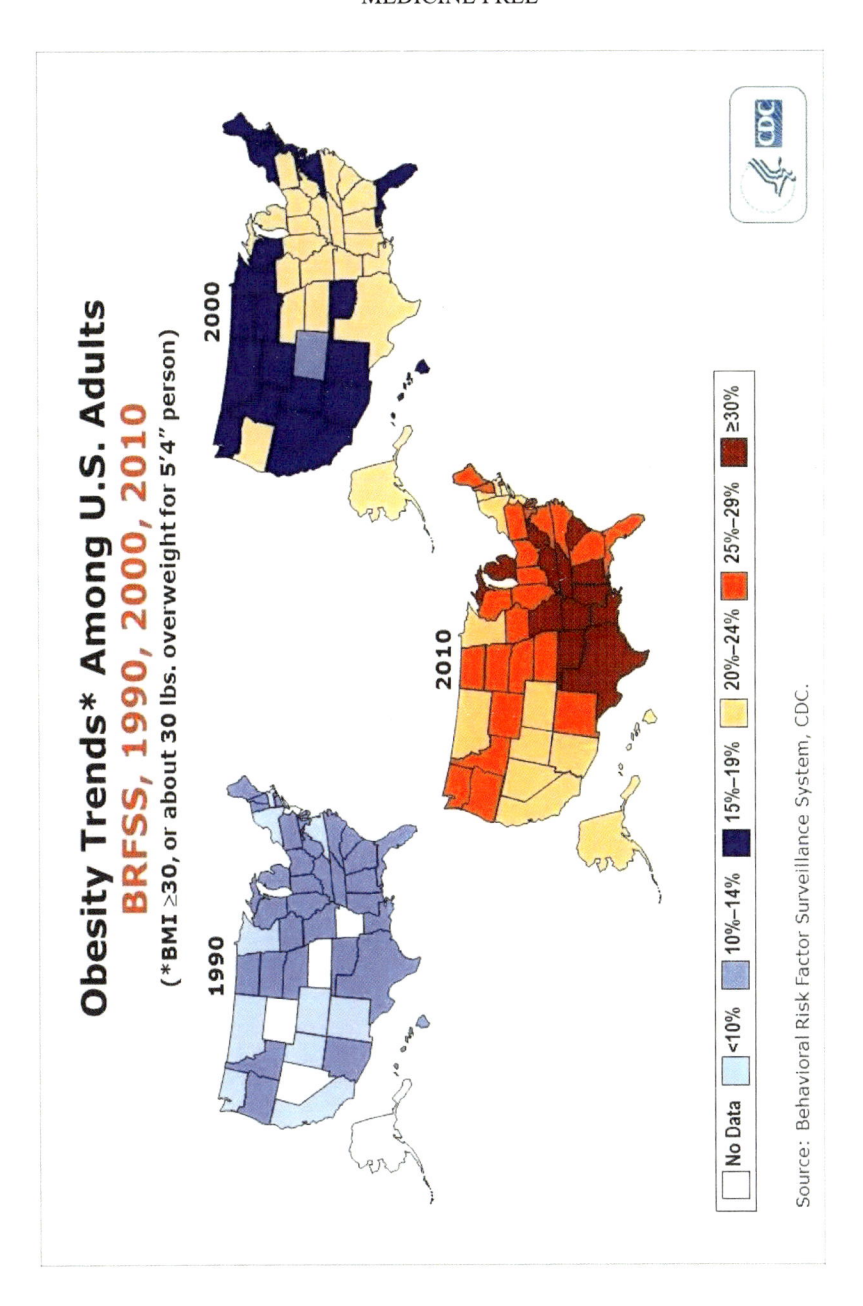

**Obesity Trends* Among U.S. Adults
BRFSS, 1990, 2000, 2010**
(*BMI ≥30, or about 30 lbs. overweight for 5'4" person)

No Data   <10%   10%–14%   15%–19%   20%–24%   25%–29%   ≥30%

Source: Behavioral Risk Factor Surveillance System, CDC.

The figure above illustrates the increased obesity rates in the United States over the last 20 years.

Dr. Bob Avery MD, FACP

Body Mass Index Table

BMI	19	20	21	22	23	24	25	26	27	28	29	30	31	32	33	34	35	36	37	38	39	40	41	42	43	44	45	46	47	48	49	50	51	52	53	54
	Normal						Overweight					Obese						Body Weight (pounds)							Extreme Obesity										
Height (inches)																																				
58	91	96	100	105	110	115	119	124	129	134	138	143	148	153	158	162	167	172	177	181	186	191	196	201	205	210	215	220	224	229	234	239	244	248	253	258
59	94	99	104	109	114	119	124	128	133	138	143	148	153	158	163	168	173	178	183	188	193	198	203	208	212	217	222	227	232	237	242	247	252	257	262	267
60	97	102	107	112	118	123	128	133	138	143	148	153	158	163	168	174	179	184	189	194	199	204	209	215	220	225	230	235	240	245	250	255	261	266	271	276
61	100	106	111	116	122	127	132	137	143	148	153	158	164	169	174	180	185	190	195	201	206	211	217	222	227	232	238	243	248	254	259	264	269	275	280	285
62	104	109	115	120	126	131	136	142	147	153	158	164	169	175	180	186	191	196	202	207	213	218	224	229	235	240	246	251	256	262	267	273	278	284	289	295
63	107	113	118	124	130	135	141	146	152	158	163	169	175	180	186	191	197	203	208	214	220	225	231	237	242	248	254	259	265	270	278	282	287	293	299	304
64	110	116	122	128	134	140	145	151	157	163	169	174	180	186	192	197	204	209	215	221	227	232	238	244	250	256	262	267	273	279	285	291	296	302	308	314
65	114	120	126	132	138	144	150	156	162	168	174	180	186	192	198	204	210	216	222	228	234	240	246	252	258	264	270	276	282	288	294	300	306	312	318	324
66	118	124	130	136	142	148	155	161	167	173	179	186	192	198	204	210	216	223	229	235	241	247	253	260	266	272	278	284	291	297	303	309	315	322	328	334
67	121	127	134	140	146	153	159	166	172	178	185	191	198	204	211	217	223	230	236	242	249	255	261	268	274	280	287	293	299	306	312	319	325	331	338	344
68	125	131	138	144	151	158	164	171	177	184	190	197	203	210	216	223	230	236	243	249	256	262	269	276	282	289	295	302	308	315	322	328	335	341	348	354
69	128	135	142	149	155	162	169	176	182	189	196	203	209	216	223	230	236	243	250	257	263	270	277	284	291	297	304	311	318	324	331	338	345	351	358	365
70	132	139	146	153	160	167	174	181	188	195	202	209	216	222	229	236	243	250	257	264	271	278	285	292	299	306	313	320	327	334	341	348	355	362	369	376
71	136	143	150	157	165	172	179	186	193	200	208	215	222	229	236	243	250	257	265	272	279	286	293	301	308	315	322	329	338	343	351	358	365	372	379	386
72	140	147	154	162	169	177	184	191	199	206	213	221	228	235	242	250	258	265	272	279	287	294	302	309	316	324	331	338	346	353	361	368	375	383	390	397
73	144	151	159	166	174	182	189	197	204	212	219	227	235	242	250	257	265	272	280	288	295	302	310	318	325	333	340	348	355	363	371	378	386	393	401	408
74	148	155	163	171	179	186	194	202	210	218	225	233	241	249	256	264	272	280	287	295	303	311	319	326	334	342	350	358	365	373	381	389	396	404	412	420
75	152	160	168	176	184	192	200	208	216	224	232	240	248	256	264	272	279	287	295	303	311	319	327	335	343	351	359	367	375	383	391	399	407	415	423	431
76	156	164	172	180	189	197	205	213	221	230	238	246	254	263	271	279	287	295	304	312	320	328	336	344	353	361	369	377	385	394	402	410	418	426	435	443

Source: Adapted from Clinical Guidelines on the Identification, Evaluation, and Treatment of Overweight and Obesity in Adults: The Evidence Report.

National Heart Lung and Blood Institute
http://www.nhlbi.nih.gov/guidelines/obesity/bmi_tbl.htm

According to the Surgeon General's report, obesity is thought to be responsible for 300,000 deaths every year in the United States and your risk of dying increases with higher weight. There is a 50-100% increased risk of death from all causes for obese individuals. Obesity is associated with a wide variety of medical conditions including heart disease, diabetes, cancer, high blood pressure, stroke, high cholesterol, sleep apnea, osteoarthritis, reproductive problems, infertility, loss of bladder control, gallbladder disease, and complications of pregnancy and surgery. According to the CDC health statistics for 2009, there are an estimated 27 million people with heart disease, 56 million with high blood pressure and 20 million with diabetes in this country. Obesity increases the risk of each of these diseases that affect a total of 103 million people or 45% of the entire U.S. population.

This is putting a large strain on the medical system in the United States. According to a report published in *USA Today* in January 2011, the cost of obesity in the United States is approaching $300 billion annually. This cost not only includes cost for health care ($127 billion) but also loss of worker productivity due to death and disability ($164 billion). These are incredible statistics since obesity is largely a preventable condition. Unfortunately, we have seen the number of obese people skyrocket over the last 20 years and we are seeing the effects on the health of this great country.

One major consequence of weight gain and obesity is metabolic syndrome. According to the Mayo Clinic, metabolic syndrome, or

Reaven's Syndrome, was first described in 1988 by Dr. Reaven from Stanford University. The syndrome primarily involves resistance to the effects of insulin. Insulin should decrease blood sugar levels but these patients were resistant to the effects. Reaven's Syndrome occurs in overweight people and was found to be a precursor to diabetes. This syndrome was later described as syndrome X and more recently as metabolic syndrome. People with metabolic syndrome characteristically are overweight and have high blood glucose level, increased blood pressure and high cholesterol levels. Weight distribution is in the center of the body so that the person is shaped like an apple not a pear. One of the easiest ways to determine if a person is at risk for metabolic syndrome is to measure their waistline. If the waistline is greater than 40 inches in men or 35 inches in women, then metabolic syndrome is likely to occur. Other findings typically found include a blood pressure of over 130/85 mmHg, a fasting blood sugar of over 100 mg/dL, and elevated cholesterol with elevated triglycerides of 150 and/or a high density lipoprotein (HDL) level of less than 40 mg/dL. Metabolic syndrome is the first step to multiple maladies including diabetes, heart disease, high blood pressure, strokes, and even cancer. It is very important and relevant because all the leading causes of disability and death are associated with metabolic syndrome.

Overeating has been thought to be the only cause of metabolic syndrome because weight gain is a major feature, but there is increasing evidence that the risk is due to other factors as well. Of course what a person eats affects their chance of gaining weight but studies also show that the diets of your mother or even grandfather also play a role. A person's diet makes epigenetic changes to their DNA which is inheritable and can be passed down to children and grandchildren. This is why it is so important to watch what you eat. It not only affects you but your descendants as well.

Observational studies on populations of women and their children have found that a mother's diet and the weight of their newborn infants will affect the baby's risk of obesity and heart disease later in life. When a woman lives in starvation conditions, her babies will be born malnourished and with a low birth weight. Paradoxically, these children have a high risk of being obese as adults. Other studies looking at infant birth weight have also demonstrated low birth weight infants have an increased risk of obesity and heart disease. The role of dietary feast or famine and their role in diseases in children were coined "thrifty genotype" and "thrifty phenotype" by Dr. Neel from the University of Michigan in 1962. Neel postulated that during times of famine certain thrifty genes were activated. These genes regulated efficient intake and storage of energy. When a child in utero is exposed to famine conditions, the thrifty genes will maximize the storage of energy. This will help them survive in a world where food is scarce. Now take this same child and feed them a diet with normal or excessive calories and the thrifty gene will lead to obesity and metabolic syndrome. In this way he accurately described what we see in real life and what scientific studies are now demonstrating.

There are other examples of maternal diet and its effect on children. We know that the risk of infant neural tube defects and congenital heart disease are higher in mothers with low folate intake.[7] This is the reason the United States and other countries supplement breads and grains with folic acid. Neural tube defects, such as spina bifida, have decreased 30-40% since folic acid has been added to grains and breads. The rate of heart defects in newborns has dropped by 45% in Canada since the institution of folic acid supplementation. Women are now instructed to take folic acid during pregnancy. The health benefits are so great that official guidelines now recommend all women who are of childbearing potential take folic acid vitamins in case they become pregnant.

The effect of the mother's diet on their child is not limited to folic acid. Children will score higher on cognitive testing if their mothers eat fish. Higher calcium intake by the mother will result in lower blood pressure in their infant, and maternal smoking is associated with low infant birth weights and an increased risk of obesity and heart disease.

The epigenetic effects of a parent's diet are not limited to children but may also affect grandchildren according to an observational study performed in Sweden. Population samples were analyzed from ancient church records. The purpose of the study was to assess the dietary intakes of grandfathers based on historical data indicating

---

[7] The neural tube is the canal where the brain and spinal cord develop. Low folate during the formation of this canal causes it to not form. The end result is the spinal cord or the brain is exposed because the bones of the back or skull do not completely form. Congenital heart defects are inherited structural defects in the heart of a baby. The heart is not formed normally resulting in problems with its ability to pump blood and deliver oxygen.

famine conditions or plentiful harvests. Food intake was assessed when the men were young boys just before puberty. Then records of the grandchildren were analyzed for the presence of heart disease. Interestingly, the risk of heart disease seemed to be affected based on what their grandfathers ate. So we see that food can have health implications for up to three generations, but as we will find out, these effects are not absolute or permanent. You can always improve your health with a healthy lifestyle. I want to show you how to change them for the better.

The question now arises, how do we think these changes occur? We are finding out that the genes themselves don't physically change, but which genes are turned on or off, do. This epigenetic mechanism is the key to health and disease and is why it is so important to have all the good genes working to be healthy.

Studies have confirmed that a mother's diet affects two key genes involved in blood sugar levels and cholesterol levels, the glucocorticoid receptor (GR) and the PPAR gene. The findings in mice demonstrated that when the mother is fed a malnutrition type of diet with low protein, both of these genes were activated leading to high blood pressure and high cholesterol levels in the offspring. The babies also had abnormal blood vessel function and early diabetes. Furthermore, the activated GR and PPAR genes were passed on to the next generation showing that a mother's diet can affect not only the health of their child but also the health of their grandchildren. This is pretty scary stuff, but another part of the research gives us hope. In the same experiment, if the mothers were supplemented with folic acid in addition to the low protein diet, the changes in the genes did not occur. You have the ability to change things for worse or better. Let's look at some examples of epigenetics in common diseases.

EPIGENETICS OF DIABETES

Diabetes Mellitus is a condition characterized by the presence of too much sugar in the blood and can occur in two ways: if there is not enough insulin produced (type I) or there is resistance to the action of insulin (type II). Under normal conditions, when the sugar level in the blood rises after a meal, the hormone insulin is released from the pancreas. Insulin causes the muscle, fat cells, and liver to remove the sugar from the blood. The sugar is then used for energy or converted to fat and stored for later use.

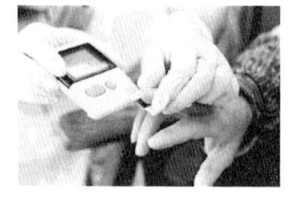

Blood sugar or glucose is the major source of energy for the body. In fact, most organisms, even bacteria, use glucose for energy. The carbohydrates in our food are converted to glucose by pancreatic enzymes. Some of the glucose is used immediately by the brain, intestinal cells and red blood cells as energy. The rest is stored as glycogen in the liver. Glycogen is a storage form that can be rapidly converted to energy, which is useful if you have to exert yourself for more than a few seconds. The cells rely on insulin in order to take up and process glucose. When the blood glucose is too high, it is filtered through the kidneys, causing the person to urinate too frequently (polyuria). This produces excessive thirst (polydipsia) and hunger (polyphagia). Polyuria, polydipsia, and polyphagia are hallmarks of diabetes.[8]

Only 5% of diabetics have type I disease, the other 95% have type II. The onset of type I disease is very rapid. A person may feel fine and then become ill over several weeks. Type II or adult onset diabetes has a very gradual onset over years. This type typically starts with metabolic syndrome and insulin resistance. The person does not even suspect the disease unless a blood test is drawn. Unfortunately, the name "adult onset" diabetes is no longer accurate because more and more children and teenagers are obese, have metabolic syndrome, and are developing diabetes.

It is estimated that 8% of adults in the United States are diagnosed with diabetes, but because of its many complications, diabetes accounts for 14% of medical expenditures. Type II diabetes tends to run in families, which suggests that it is inherited, while Type I diabetes is not

---

[8] The word diabetes is derived from the Greek word which means siphon or passing through in reference to the polyuria. This was described by the ancient Greek physician Areteus of Cappadocia who lived in the first Century B.C. The word Mellitus was attached to the name by Thomas Willis, a 17th Century English physician. Mellitus is the Latin word for honey and was a description of the sweet taste of the urine in diabetics. Yes, in the 17th Century it would be common practice or the physician to taste the urine if this disease was suspected. Areteus, who is known for his works on the description of disease was the first to characterize the intense thirst and urination in patients with this disease. He also wrote "the disease consists in a waste of the flesh, and solution of different parts of the body into urine" referring to the loss of weight found in patients with type I diabetes. This was a devastating disease because there was no treatment available until the development of insulin for injection in 1920. Thereafter, the disease has been easier to manage.

inherited. There are many genes involved in diabetes; environment and diet play a key role in the cause and prevention. What you eat is not only the cause of diabetes, it can be the cure.

A diabetic's chronically elevated blood sugar causes an increase in oxidation and inflammation of the blood vessels, lipids and proteins. The lining of blood vessels, or the endothelium, is very important for regulation of the blood, blood pressure, and the clotting system. In people without diabetes, oxidation is normally controlled by antioxidant enzymes and nutrients, but the level of oxidation in a diabetic is so high it overwhelms the system and chronically damages proteins and blood vessels. This damage leads to an increased risk of atherosclerotic disease and abnormal blood clotting. The result is heart disease, heart attacks and strokes which are common diseases in people with advanced diabetes.

Recent studies have demonstrated how diabetes causes medical problems through changes in gene expression. Even temporary increases in blood sugars can change gene expression. Short periods of high blood sugar alter specific genes which lead to increased inflammation. The bad news is these altered genes and inflammation remain even after the blood sugar is normalized in an effect called metabolic memory or a legacy effect and it highlights the importance of preventing a disease before it becomes advanced. In large studies of diabetic patients randomized to either control tightly or loose control of their blood sugar, there was no difference in the rate of heart attacks based on how well the sugar was controlled. It is thought that the damage had been done early on in the disease; changing the blood sugar level later had little effect. The authors attributed the findings to the legacy effect. Inflammatory genes were altered and remained damaged even if the blood sugar was normalized.

This does not mean that treatment of diabetes is pointless or not worth trying. These studies were only looking at controlling blood sugar levels with insulin and its effect on complications of the disease. The study did not specifically address lifestyle issues, only blood sugar levels. In my opinion, the rate of heart attacks did not decrease primarily because the patient's diet was not improved. Controlling the blood sugar with insulin does not negate the inflammation and oxidation produced by a poor diet. In my mind, the diet is a necessary factor in preventing complications from diabetes.

We know that diet plays a key role in diabetes, especially energy sources and carbohydrates. There are simple carbohydrates such as sugars, glucose, fructose, and there are complex carbohydrates, such as starches, from grains. Foods with carbohydrates will elevate the blood sugar after you eat them. The glycemic index is a measure of how high your blood sugar is elevated after you eat 50 grams of a particular carbohydrate. A larger glycemic index number indicates a higher rise in blood sugar. Glycemic load takes into account the serving size of the food. Some foods with high glycemic indexes, such as carrots, have a low glycemic load because the serving size of one carrot does not have a lot of carbohydrates. Foods with high glycemic indexes and glycemic loads will lead to metabolic syndrome and diabetes. They also make the diabetes difficult to control if they remain in the patient's diet.

In the past, diabetics were told to avoid simple carbohydrates and eat more complex carbohydrates because of the assumption that they would be more beneficial for blood sugar. This was a simple formula, avoid sugars and eat more bread and pasta. As it turns out, this was too simplistic. Glycemic index levels reveal that even complex carbohydrates can be detrimental to your blood sugar level. To make things more difficult, the glycemic index is not only affected by the amount of sugars and starch, but also by the amount of fat, protein, and fiber in the foods you eat. Here are some of the factors that can alter the glycemic index of a particular food:

1. Ripeness: The riper a fruit or vegetable is, the higher the GI.

2. Processing: Fruit juice has a higher GI than whole fruit, mashed potatoes than baked potato, bread with processed flour compared to stone ground grains in bread.

3. Cooking method: al dente pasta has a lower GI than overcooked, soft pasta

4. Variety: long grain and brown rice has a lower GI than short grain white rice.

5. Other ingredients: fiber and fat content will lower the GI of foods.

There is now evidence to show high carbohydrate, not high fat, diets lead to obesity. In the past, high fat diets were once thought to be the source of the obesity epidemic in America. Recommendations from major health organizations like the U.S. Government Department of

Health and Human Services (1988), the American Heart Association (1996), and the American Diabetes Association (1997) suggested a low fat diet was necessary to prevent obesity. This concept has been questioned by several investigators, and although the fat content in the American diet has fallen from 42% in the 1960's to 34% in the 1990's, we have seen an incredible increase in the number of obese persons in the United States. It seems clear that fat content in the diet is not to blame for the American weight problem.

Although protein content has remained relatively stable in diets over the last decades, there has been an increase in carbohydrate content in the American diet since the 1970's due to an increase in low-fat dieting. When a person eats a low fat diet, the higher fat foods are usually replaced by a menu of carbohydrates. The problem with this is twofold. First, the carbohydrates selected by a person on a low fat diet tend to have a high GI and there is less fat to slow stomach absorption. One benefit of dietary fat is digestion is slowed and as a result, the glycemic index also falls. Any carbohydrate paired with a low fat meal is higher on the GI index then without the fat.

Don't calories in equal calories out? No. Why would more weight gain occur with carbohydrate calories than fat calories? The answer appears to be insulin. As you recall, insulin is the hormone that drives blood sugar into the liver and fat cells. High glycemic index carbohydrates not only raise the blood sugar but also insulin levels. The insulin level is raised higher by high glycemic index foods than lower glycemic index foods of equal calories. Higher insulin levels lead to increased fat deposition. We know this from treating diabetics. Patients with Type I diabetes have a lack of insulin production and have profound weight loss before diagnosis. Insulin treatment then not only lowers the blood sugar but also causes weight gain. Similar findings of weight gain are found in Type II diabetics if they are given insulin as therapy. So the old adage of "calories in = calories out" is not correct. The source of the calorie is important. In terms of weight control, lower glycemic index foods are more beneficial than high glycemic index foods. High-fat or protein diets can actually lead to weight loss as long as the carbohydrates and glycemic index are low. We'll find out more about how low carbohydrate diets can affect your weight and your health later in the book.

EPIGENETICS OF HEART DISEASE

The heart is the most important organ in the body. Its function is to pump blood. The heart beats an average of 72 times per minute and 100,000 times per day. Approximately 1.3 gallons of blood pass through the heart every minute, 1,900 gallons per day and 700,000 gallons each year. That is a lot of work and to do it, the heart muscle must be kept healthy through diet and exercise. If not, heart disease develops.

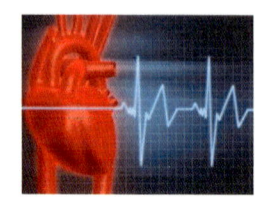

Heart disease is the number one cause of death in America. Every year approximately 615,000 people die of heart attacks, 440,000

of them die of sudden cardiac death before reaching the hospital, and over 1.2 million people have a heart attack every year. Heart disease comes in many forms. There can be problems with the muscle or pump function, the valves, the heart rhythm, or the blood vessels. Disease of the blood vessels has several names including atherosclerosis, arteriosclerosis, and hardening of the arteries. The basic problem is a buildup of calcified plaques inside the blood vessels. Gradually, the plaques block off the artery and decrease the blood flow to the heart muscle. This causes the heart muscle to cramp, which is called angina. Angina can be mild and occur only with strenuous exercise, or it can be very severe and occur at a resting heart rate. If and when the plaque ruptures, it causes a blood clot to form on the area which can completely block the artery. Without blood flow, the muscle dies. This is a heart attack.

The risk factors for heart disease include male gender, increasing age, high blood pressure, high blood cholesterol, diabetes, tobacco, obesity, physical inactivity, and family history. All of these risk factors can be modified except for your gender, age and family history.

You can't change your family's history of heart disease but you can change your risk of disease, even if you have inherited one of the genes that have been identified as a gene that leads to heart disease.[9] The ninth chromosome is strongly influential. Abnormalities on the ninth chromosome are associated with a 30% increase in the risk of heart

---

[9] There are approximately 30 locations on different chromosomes that have a role in the development of heart disease. The abnormalities in the gene location 9p21 are associated with a 30% increase in the risk of heart attacks.

disease. A study in Europe examined people with abnormalities on the ninth chromosome, observing their risk of heart attack while on a diet high in raw fruits and vegetables. As it turned out, those who ate a diet high in raw fruits and vegetables decreased the risk of heart attack by 30%. This is the same risk level seen in people without the abnormal gene. This is an excellent example of how lifestyle can trump a bad gene and improve the risk of heart attacks.

Overall, there has been a decrease in heart related mortality over the last 30 years due to improved therapies such as coronary bypass, heart stents and medical therapies; but don't discount the importance of improved lifestyle. We too often fall into the trap of relying on technologies, such as bypass surgery or angioplasty to treat our heart disease, and discount the benefits of a healthful lifestyle which decreases the risk of dying from heart disease. There has been a 31% decrease in heart disease and heart attacks in women over the last 15 years due to reduced smoking, improved diet, and discontinuing hormone replacement therapy. This trend should continue as smoking rates decrease every year. Unfortunately, not every demographic group in the U.S. is following a prudent diet. A person has an 80% greater chance of having heart disease if they grow up in an underprivileged area. Persons in this environment are more likely to be overweight, eat bad foods, use tobacco, have high blood pressure, and high cholesterol. However, if these risk factors are removed, the risk of heart disease drops significantly, demonstrating that it's not too late to develop good habits whenever possible. A healthy lifestyle will lead to better health.

The most harmful lifestyle choice people make today is to smoke tobacco. Tobacco smoke is loaded with cancer-causing chemicals and also leads to oxidative damage of proteins, DNA, and blood vessels. Tobacco has also been demonstrated to cause changes in gene methylation whether we are exposed in the womb or as adult smokers. These data show clearly how powerful tobacco smoke is in changing our genes and leading to an increased risk of heart disease and cancer. There is some data to suggest that certain foods like broccoli and cauliflower can help protect you from the effects of tobacco, but quitting tobacco is always the best option. I ask my patients "if you hit your head with a hammer, you get a concussion. If you wear a helmet it might take a few more hits of the hammer to give you a concussion, but isn't it better not to hit your head in the first place?" So why are you still smoking?

We have seen the effects of epigenetics on your risk of heart disease. What your parents or grandparents ate can affect your health, but you don't have to resign yourself to their legacy. Studies are showing that good lifestyle choices can change your genes and your risk of heart disease. If we've learned anything from the study of epigenetics, it's that many of these changes can be reversed with lifestyle.

EPIGENETICS OF CANCER

Cancer is the second leading cause of death in men and women in the United States. What exactly is a cancer? A cancer is abnormal growth of cells that may form from any tissue in the body: lung, colon, breast, muscle, brain, or bone marrow to name a few, and these cancers cause problems in multiple ways. They directly destroy tissues by invasion or can spread throughout the body (metastasis). Cancer cells do not function as normal cells do, so cancers of the immune cells such as leukemia or lymphoma do not fight infections normally. This leads to an increased risk of infection. Finally, advanced cancers affect the body's metabolism leading to loss of appetite, loss of weight, fatigue and debility. Unfortunately, most everyone has seen the effects of cancer in a loved one. Early on in the disease, the person may look perfectly well, but there is no mistaking the devastating effects later on.

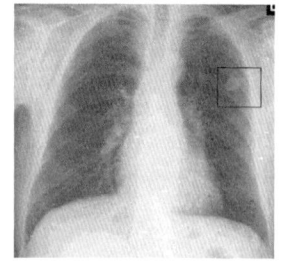

There have been a lot of theories about the cause of cancer. Centuries ago it was thought to be caused by black bile. In the past century, it was thought that infections or trauma caused cancer. It wasn't until the last 20 years that cancer causing genes were discovered. The first cancer causing genes, or oncogenes, were discovered in 1989. Today we know of several inherited cancer genes that lead to breast, colon, kidney and other cancers, but these are the minority of cancer cases. For example, the breast cancer genes BRCA-1 and BRCA-2 are only responsible for 7% of breast cancer cases overall. It is becoming clear that the majority of cancers, like heart disease and diabetes, are due to lifestyle choices and epigenetics.

The majority of research in epigenetics is from cancer research.

It has been known for 30 years that cancer cells have an abnormal amount of methylation. In general, cancers cells have low levels of methyl groups, but locally increased levels of methyl groups. Remember, methyl groups are the chemical off switch for genes. The areas with low methylation are in areas where cancer causing genes exist, while the high-level methylation areas are responsible for turning off tumor suppressing genes. There is also data to show that there is abnormal activity in histones – the spools the DNA is wound around. Currently we know epigenetics plays a role in breast, colon, lung, brain, bladder, kidney, prostate, esophagus, stomach, liver, lymphoma and ovarian cancers.

The knowledge of this connection between cancer and epigenetics is vitally important. Can you change your risk of cancer even if you have a family history of cancer? Yes. You can change your genes and affect your risk by making simple lifestyle choices. A diet high in fruits and vegetables, good fats, and low in red meat – especially processed meat – will help turn on all the processes and genes in your body that will prevent cancer. Studies have shown you will decrease your risk by up to 50%. Now I will show you how you can improve your health on a daily basis. It's not difficult, just keep reading.

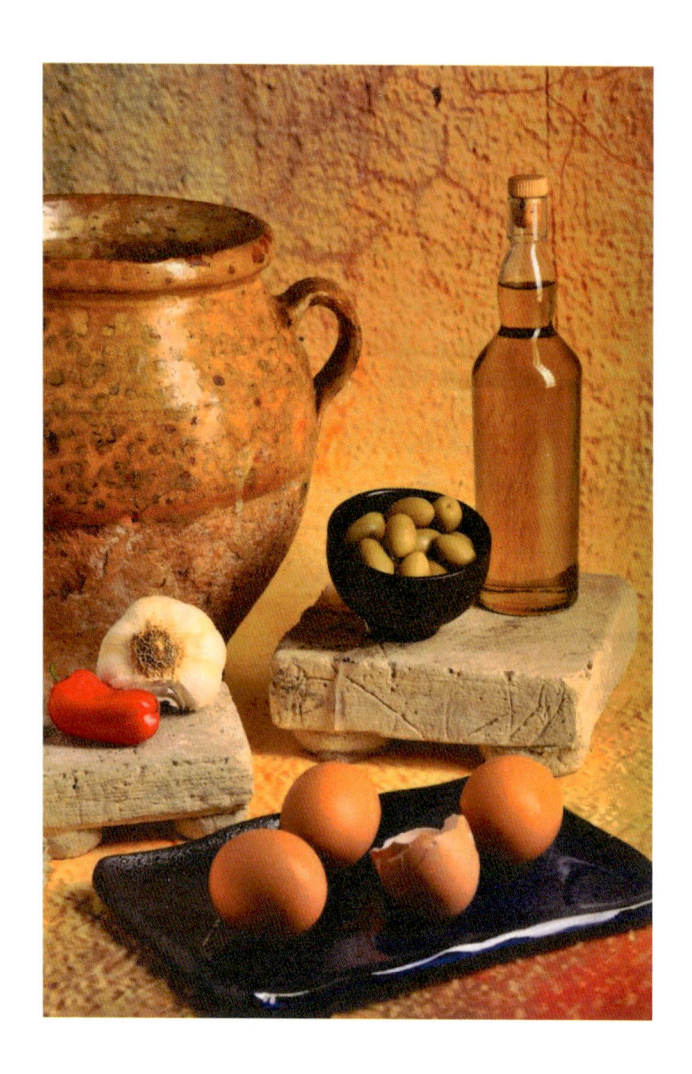

2. NUTRIGENOMICS-Natural Healing

We have discussed how epigenetics affects your health.[10] Now we know that most diseases are caused by poor lifestyle choices, poor diet, lack of nutrition, or lack of exercise, leading to abnormal expression of genes through epigenetic changes. Up until this point in the book, we have concentrated on the cause of disease without studying what can be done to prevent or reverse it. Now we can discuss how you can prevent or reverse diseases.

One criticism of modern Western medicine is it treats the symptoms of diseases but not the causes. Medicines for high blood pressure will bring the blood pressure down effectively, but the moment you stop the medicine, the blood pressure will increase again. Wouldn't it be better to not have high blood pressure in the first place, free from the burden of the disease and the expense of treating it? Of course, it's easier said than done. There will always be people who don't want to change their lifestyle to be healthy, instead looking to pills to fix the problem.

Physicians, on the other hand, find it too easy just to prescribe a pill instead of spending time to change patient attitudes and habits. It also gives the impression that medicine and pharmaceutical companies are only interested in treating diseases rather than curing them. This

---

[10] Genes are turned off by methylation or turned on by removing methyl groups. We also discussed how the DNA in our cells is wound around a spool called a histone. When an acetyl group is added to the histone, it loosens its grip on the DNA and the strand unwinds. This allows the genes to be activated. Enzymes called histone de-acetylases remove the acetyl group and the DNA winds tight. No genes are activated in this situation.

approach to illness has helped the pharmaceutical industry grow into the 26th highest grossing industry in the United States with an annual income of $315 billion in 2009. It is in their best interest, not yours, if you keep taking pills to tackle poor health and disease.

Can high blood pressure – the major cause of heart disease and stroke – be treated without medicines? The answer is yes. The first step in treating anyone with high blood pressure is to alter his or her lifestyle. Increasing exercise, weight loss and cutting salt intake are very effective in lowering blood pressure. Weight loss of only 5 pounds will begin to drop blood pressure, and those who lose 20 pounds or more can drop their blood pressure an average of 8 points. Weight loss through either dieting or gastric bypass surgery is beneficial. A person who loses significant weight by either means will not only drop his blood pressure, but will also improve his glucose intolerance and lower blood sugars even if he is considered pre-diabetic. Low vitamin D has been found to cause high blood pressure and is a risk factor for heart disease. Several studies have also shown that taking a vitamin D supplement can drop the blood pressure 5-7 points on average. So, natural treatments for diseases do exist and we can reverse disease without medications. How do you think this works? You're right, through epigenetics.

The Agouti Mouse: proof that food can turn off genes

The story of the Agouti gene in mice is fascinating and really highlights the power of food and nutrition over our genes. The Agouti gene controls the distribution of black pigment in coats of animals. When the Agouti gene is turned off in horses, they have a uniform black pigment. The Agouti gene affects the color of the coat in mice as well, resulting in yellow mice when it is active, but it also has other physiologic effects: the yellow mice are also overweight, prone to chronic diseases and have a shortened lifespan. The Agouti gene, like all genes, is passed from one generation to the next, so the offspring will also be yellow and fat.

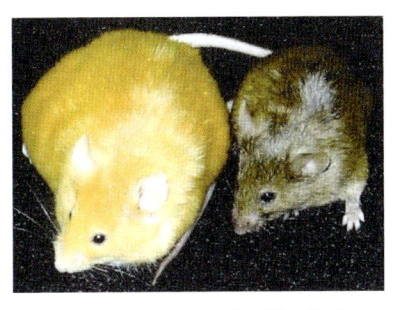

Published with permission, Dr. Jirtle

Researchers out of Duke University performed a simple, but elegant experiment. We know that genes are turned off by attaching a methyl group at the starting point for the gene, so they studied the effect of diet on the agouti gene. First, they put the female yellow mice on a methyl donor diet consisting of onions, garlic and beets. They also ensured that the mice had an adequate supply of vitamin B12, choline, and betaine in their diet. This maximized their ability to produce methyl groups to transfer to the DNA.

After the yellow mice had been on this diet for a sufficient period of time, they were allowed to breed. What happened was astonishing. The methyl groups found their way into the DNA of the fetus and turned off the Agouti gene. These pups had dark coats, were normal in appearance, were not overweight, and had a normal lifespan. So with a simple change in diet, these researchers demonstrated that the undesirable gene could be turned off. This finding is especially important for us, since we all have bad genes in our bodies; but we can control our diet to influence their behavior for the better.

HEALTHFUL BENEFITS OF SPECIFIC FOODS:

Which foods are the best for us to eat? Generally we can say fruits and vegetables, fish, good carbs and good fats. But why are these particular foods considered healthful? We are now finding out that many of these foods have epigenetic effects by changing our genes and making us healthier. The study of how food nutrients change genes is called *nutrigenomics*. The fields of epigenetics and nutrigenomics are very exciting but still young and we have much more to learn. Every food will have a nutrigenomic effect, we just haven't had time to study every food in existence yet. Here is a list of some of the most studied foods and their nutrigenomic effects.

Green tea:

Next to water, tea is the most popular drink in the world. Tea has a rich and diverse history. Its earliest recorded use was in China in the 10th Century B.C. In China, tea serves as a drink for ceremonies as well as a medicine for a variety of ailments. Tea has been used as a stimulant due to its caffeine content, for respiratory ailments due to its theophylline content, and for general gastrointestinal afflictions.

Although there are many forms of tea (white, yellow, green, black, and oolong), every form is made from the same *Camellia sinensis* plant. Different varieties of tea are produced by altering the way in which the leaves are processed. The *Camellia Sinensis* is an evergreen plant that grows in tropical and subtropical areas, but some varieties tolerate cooler climates and are grown as far north as Washington State. If left alone, the plants grow to a height of 50 feet, but to assist in harvesting, they are pruned to waist height. Only the youngest leaves from the top 1-2 inches of the plant are harvested for tea. Soon after the leaf is picked it begins to wilt and oxidize as enzymes break down the chlorophyll inside the leaves. As this happens, the leaves darken and turn black producing black tea. The oxidation process can be stopped at any time by heating the leaves to 160 degrees. Heating the leaves immediately produces green tea.

Tea, like many fruits and vegetables, contains organic compounds called polyphenols. Much of its health benefits are attributed to polyphenols. The polyphenol compound in tea leaves is called epigallocatechin 3-gallate or EGCG. It is the most abundant phenol in tea, especially green tea. EGCG increases the production of antioxidant enzymes and is an excellent antioxidant. The benefits of tea, especially the heart benefits have been thought to be due to the antioxidant effects, but recent research reveals much more about EGCG.

There are many beneficial actions of green tea and EGCG. EGCG is anti-inflammatory, antibacterial, anti-oxidation, anti-viral, it protects nerves, lowers cholesterol, and helps with weight reduction. People who drink green tea regularly have a decrease risk of heart disease and cancer. As you can see, EGCG has benefits all over your body. Let's investigate the healthy benefits of tea in more detail.

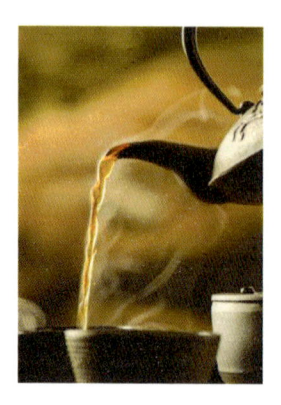

Tea and Heart Health

The complex cardiovascular system is based on component systems: muscles, blood vessels, cholesterol, and platelet function. These are affected by oxidation and inflammation. Many, if not all of these, are positively affected by green tea and the EGCG it contains. EGCG is an anti-oxidant, and both decreases inflammation and helps to improve cholesterol levels. EGCG helps to prevent growth of smooth muscle cells, which is important to prevent narrowing of blood vessels and blockage of heart stents. Finally, EGCG suppresses platelet function, which helps to prevent heart attacks.

Tea and Cancer

Animal models have suggested green tea can prevent many different types of cancer including skin, lung, mouth/throat, esophageal, stomach, liver, pancreas, small intestine, colon, bladder, prostate, and breast. There are many ways in which green tea prevents or inhibits cancers. First, it has been shown to decrease the formation of cancers in animals after exposure to a cancer-causing chemical (carcinogen). EGCG will also cause cancer cells to die through a process called programmed cell death. Finally, EGCG is an inhibitor of DNA methyltransferase which has the effect of removing methyl groups from the promoter regions of genes, allowing tumor-suppressing genes to be activated.

When EGCG is added to cultures of head and neck tumor cells in lab conditions, it inhibits the action of several growth factors and their receptors. This includes the growth factor for cell growth (epidermal growth factor) and the factor for blood vessel growth (vascular endothelial growth factor). Without growth factor stimulation, the tumor cells simply will not develop and grow. In esophageal cancer cells, EGCG was found to remove the methyl groups from the tumor-suppressing genes, allowing them to function normally. Studies in humans show that green tea can reverse pre-cancerous patches in the mouth, precancerous cervix lesions, and prevent the development of prostate cancer.

Other Benefits of Tea

A recent review in the Chinese Medical Journal outlined the wide range of other possible benefits of tea: prevention of chronic disease, protection of the liver, lowering cholesterol, immune system modulation, neurologic disorders, and weight loss. Tea polyphenols, especially those from green tea, have multiple health benefits. Incorporating tea into your diet plan would be very beneficial.

Caution: Don't Drink Too Much Tea

Most studies show that drinking three to seven cups of tea in a week are beneficial, but too much tea can be harmful. Tea contains fluoride, which can cause brittle bones at high levels. Fluoride will increase the bone mineral density of your bones, but that does not protect them from fracture. It actually makes them brittle and easier to break. Tea also contains aluminum, which is harmful to the bones and brain in large doses - especially if you have kidney problems. Tea contains oxalate, which will prevent the absorption of iron from the diet and lead to iron deficiency. Additionally, pregnant or nursing women are advised not to drink more than one to two cups of tea daily because of the caffeine content.

Grapes:

Grapes are a berry that grows on vines and are found all over the world. Grapes can be eaten raw or made into juice, jams, jelly, vinegar, wine, raisins or molasses. Grapes come in two varieties: table grapes or wine grapes. One of the most common products of grapes is wine. The art of making wine dates back to 4000 B.C. in Persia. Wine has occupied a prominent position in cultures since that time. In fact, wine was considered a drink of the gods by ancient Greeks and Romans. More recently, research has identified many health benefits of grapes and wine.

It's been known for years that drinking moderate amounts of wine may decrease the risk of heart disease and heart attacks. The country most famous for demonstrating this benefit is France. The French eat a diet that contains as much as 16% saturated fat, but in spite of this high fat diet, the rate of heart attacks and cardiac mortality in France is only 25% of the rate of Northern Europe. The difference has been attributed to drinking wine. This association is so impressive it has been called the "French Paradox".

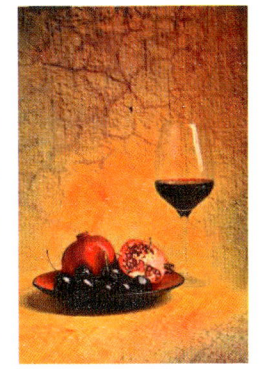

Grapes have many health benefits thanks to the powerful nutrients they contain; they decrease oxidation, slow aging, and help prevent cancers. The skin of the grape is especially healthy because it is loaded with polyphenols similar to those in tea. The most studied phenol in grapes is resveratrol; like other polyphenols, it has healthy nutrigenomic effects. Clearly, if you really study their diet, the real secret ingredient behind the French Paradox is resveratrol. How does resveratrol's anti-aging, anti-cancer, and heart-healthful magic work? Let's find out.

There are many ways resveratrol and other polyphenols prevent atherosclerosis. They inhibit oxidation of LDL cholesterol, prevent platelet activation, regulate smooth muscle growth in blood vessels and increase production of nitric oxide, which helps relax blood vessels and prevent blood clots. Grapes also contain pterostilbine, a form of resveratrol, which has been found to lower bad cholesterol levels by activating a gene in the liver that is responsible for regulating blood cholesterol. It affects all three systems associated with heart disease: oxidized lipids, overactive platelets and abnormal blood vessels. This makes resveratrol one of the most healthful nutrients for the heart.

Resveratrol also inhibits cancer cells from growing. It does this through a variety of mechanisms. First, through a plant form of estrogen called a phytoestrogen, resveratrol is able to inhibit hormone sensitive cancers like prostate cancer and breast cancer. Prostate cancer cells will stop producing DNA and stop growing in the presence of resveratrol. Breast cancer cells also stop growing because resveratrol changes the methyl groups on the genes. Resveratrol also helps maintain the activity of the breast cancer gene BRCA. Under normal conditions, the BRCA gene helps to repair DNA but when mutated, it is associated with an aggressive form of hereditary breast cancer. Further studies have shown resveratrol inhibits cancer formation in all phases: formation, growth, and metastatic spread.

Does Resveratrol Help You Live Longer?

If you consider its heart health and anticancer benefits, the answer is yes, but there is more to the story. In tests on animal diet and lifespan, an animal on restricted intake of 50% fewer calories than normal will live 50% longer than a similar animal on full caloric intake. This is true in multiple species. The mechanism behind the increased life span is an epigenetic change in the DNA. Calorie restriction causes activation of sirtuins. Sirtuins are histone deacetylases; they remove acetyl groups from histones – the spool DNA is wound around. This tightens the grip the histone has on the DNA and winds the DNA tight. In this tightened state, the genes in the DNA are silent. Deacetylation also seems to activate processes involved in the repair of DNA mutations. This is the likely mechanism to the benefits seen with sirtuin activation. So what do grapes have to do with these processes? Grapes contain resveratrol; resveratrol activates sirtuins, which has been shown to increase the life span of animals. Studies in humans have not yet been completed so we don't know if this effect can be reproduced in you and me. Nonetheless, grapes are still great for your health.

Flaxseed:

Flaxseed is a seed from the plant *Linum usitatissimum,* which is harvested for its seeds and oil. The plant can also be used to produce linen. Flaxseed is one of the first crops to be domesticated and it has long been used in medicine. Some of the historical uses of flaxseed include treatment of bowel disorders (such as constipation or irritable bowel syndrome), inflammation, heart disease, acne, ADHD, lupus, menopausal symptoms, breast pain, sore throat and upper respiratory illnesses. The Natural Medicines Comprehensive Database, which bases its recommendations on scientific evidence, lists the probable benefits of flaxseed as lowering blood sugar in diabetics, lowering cholesterol in people with high cholesterol, improving kidney function in people with systemic lupus, and relieving mild menopausal symptoms.

One beneficial component of flaxseed is lignin, which is a phytoestrogen, which has been found to slow the growth rate of prostate cancer cells in men prior to having prostate cancer surgery. Lignin also inhibits the growth promoting effects of estrogen on breast cancer cells. Heart disease can be positively affected by flaxseed as well. It inhibits the formation of atherosclerotic plaques in the blood vessels and, at higher doses, inhibits inflammation.

Green Leafy Vegetables:

Green leafy vegetables are some of the most nutritious vegetables we can eat. Spinach, kale, collards, turnip greens, Swiss chard, mustard greens, and the wide variety of lettuces are classified as green leafy vegetables. They are nutrition powerhouses and should be included in your diet every day. Some of the multitude of nutrients found in green leafy vegetables include vitamin A (especially lutein), carotenes (especially zeaxanthin), folate, vitamin C, vitamin K, vitamin E, B vitamins, magnesium, manganese, iron, betaine, calcium, potassium, copper, selenium, phosphorus, zinc, and niacin. A diet high in green leafy vegetables has been associated with a decreased risk of heart disease, stroke, cancer, macular degeneration, Alzheimer's disease, and Type II diabetes.

Their biologic effects are many. Green leafy vegetables contain nutrients like folate that are necessary for the production of DNA, and the growth of cells, like red blood cells. There are antioxidant and anti-inflammatory nutrients. There are nutrients like betaine and folate that are necessary to make DNA and to generate methyl groups to regulate genes. The carotenes, including lutein and zeaxanthin, have been found to help prevent diseases of the eye, including macular degeneration, and they are linked to the prevention of cancers and heart disease. Carotenoids not only act as antioxidants but they also enhance the repair of DNA. Isothiocyanates in kale help prevent cancer. Green leafy vegetables contain nearly every nutrient you need to live a healthy life. Go Green!

Tomato:

The tomato was once thought to be poisonous and is often misclassified as a vegetable. Far from being either, it is a tasty fruit that comes in a wide variety of types and is a food staple in the United States. The red color of the tomato comes from a phytochemical called lycopene. This chemical substance has received a lot of attention from researchers because of its health benefits.

Lycopene is in the class of carotenoids and is found in tomatoes, carrots, watermelons, and papayas. Eating tomatoes has been shown to decrease the risk of chronic diseases, heart disease and cancer. Lycopene is a powerful antioxidant, able to scavenge free oxygen radicals and prevent damage to DNA, proteins, and lipids. There are convincing studies demonstrating a decreased level of oxidized LDL cholesterol after only one week's supplementation with lycopene. Tomato juice, an excellent source of lycopene, also will decrease oxidized LDL, as will tomato puree. Since oxidized LDL is a major risk factor for heart disease, we can expect tomatoes will help reduce atherosclerosis and heart disease.

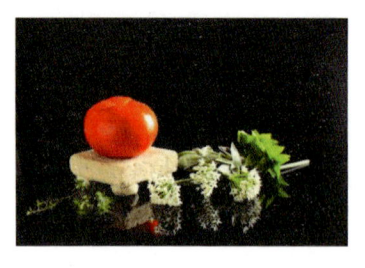

There are other beneficial effects of lycopene in addition to its antioxidant actions. Lycopene has been shown to inhibit the growth of several different types of cancer cells including prostate, breast, colon, lung and uterine. Lycopene can also modestly drop the LDL cholesterol level, as much as 14% in one study. The mechanism of action is actually the same as the commonly prescribed medicines called statins. Lycopene inhibits the same enzyme, HMGCoA reductase, that statin medicines such as Lipitor, Crestor, and Pravachol do. Amazing, foods can actually work the same way medicines do! Why not let food be your medicine?

Cruciferous vegetables:

Cruciferous vegetables include broccoli, cauliflower, cabbage, Brussels sprouts, Bok choi, kale, arugula, horse radish, wasabi, watercress, rutabaga, and turnips. They are the gas-producing vegetables so they aren't the most socially acceptable vegetables to serve at a dinner party, but they have some incredible health benefits!

The active agents in cruciferous vegetables are isothyocyanates, including sulforaphane and Indole-3-Carbinole, which have been found to prevent cancer by a variety of means.

Cancer-causing chemicals, also called carcinogens, can be found everywhere, even in what we eat or drink. Carcinogens include pesticides, herbicides, or nitrosamines in grilled meat or tobacco. Fortunately, there have been many studies demonstrating the ability of cruciferous vegetables to help detoxify our food by causing the production of enzymes that eat up carcinogens. The sulforaphane found in these vegetables slows the growth of cancer cells and causes them to die. It also works as a histone deacetylase inhibitor, like resveratrol, tightening up DNA and increasing DNA repair mechanisms. Studies on isothyocyanates also have demonstrated that they protect cell DNA from damage from tobacco smoke and harness the oxidation system to kill cancer cells directly. There doesn't seem to be anything a cruciferous vegetable can't do.

NATURAL HEALING:

How Nutrition Helps your Stem Cells and the Immune System

How do you heal yourself? So far we have discussed how nutrition can help change genes and prevent or reverse disease, but how do we use this information in a practical way? The healing cells in your body are stem cells and the immune system. Stem cells have received much media attention because of their use to treat diseases. Adult stem cells have been used successfully to treat a variety of diseases such as cancer, and they show potential promise for other conditions like heart disease and stroke. Embryonic stem cells are also being studied in a variety of diseases. Did you know that you have your own stem cells? They serve a very important purpose: repair and replacement of damaged tissues. Let's look a little closer at what a stem cell is and how we can harness our own stem cells.

Stem cells are the first cells present when life begins. At fertilization, the egg and sperm combine into a single cell containing the genes from both the mother and father. This one cell is the first stem cell and it has the potential to become any cell in the body. Eventually, it will transform into all the cells that make up the fully formed embryo. The ability to become any other cell in the body is called pluripotency and this ability distinguishes stem cells from other cells.

Forming a baby is not the only function of a stem cell, however. Once we are fully formed, we still need stem cells to repair or replace tissues, especially in organs where cells don't live very long. Each cell in our body has a defined life expectancy depending on the type of organ. Red blood cells live 120 days, white blood cells live up to 3 days, colon cells live 3-4 days, pancreas cells live 1 year or more, and brain cells live our entire life. Stem cells in the gut and bone marrow are highly active because of the short life span of those cells. In other organs, such as the brain, pancreas, or heart, cell turnover is infrequent. The stem cells are needed only under situations when these tissues are damaged and need repair, such as a stroke or heart attack.

Our tissues do not contain many stem cells, which makes them difficult to find and difficult to study. Stem cells were once thought to live only in the bone marrow (where they are called mesenchymal stem cells). Over the years, however, they have been found in virtually every other tissue, including the dental pulp, lining of the uterus, amniotic fluid, umbilical cord, fat tissues, bone and blood vessels. Stems cells do not exist alone but live in small communities called niches composed of tissue cells, supporting matrix tissues, growth factors and hormones. All of the components of the niche influence the function and type of cell the stem cell will become. For instance, if a stem cell is placed in a stomach niche, it becomes a stomach cell and not a bone cell. Likewise, if you put a stem cell in heart tissue, it will become a heart cell. Current stem cell research is trying to take advantage of this replacement process by injecting stem cells directly into damaged tissue in hopes that the stem cells will replace the damaged cells. In the future, this will be a fantastic treatment for people who have had a heart attack or stroke.

A specific characteristic of stem cells is their ability to regenerate. When they divide, they produce more stem cells that have no defined life span. Once a stem cell becomes committed to becoming a specific type of cell, however, it will have the characteristics and life span of that cell. As we age, our stem cells lose the ability to regenerate, which means that we have fewer stem cells available to repair damaged cells. Many of the changes we see with aging can be attributed to a decline in stem cell function. Not surprisingly, stem cells have become important in the study of aging and disease.

Studies of the aging process have found many changes in aging stem cells. In our tissues, aging is associated with a decrease in the number of stem cells as well as a decrease in stem function. Stem cells, like other cells, can be damaged by inflammation and oxidation. These mutate the DNA directly or cause epigenetic changes in the DNA affecting the ability of the stem cells to function normally. This decline in stem cell function is described as stem cell exhaustion. If you imagine the stem cells constantly working to repair or replace damaged tissues, it makes sense that eventually they can become burned out from battling poor diet, smoking, alcohol, inflammation and oxidation. Research has demonstrated metabolic syndrome, with its associated inflammation and oxidation, decreases stem number and function. This has been found to accelerate the course of the resulting heart disease because there are fewer stem cells to help repair the damage. You can see now how poor lifestyle choices lead to premature aging by damaging your stem cells. The key to a long, healthy life is preserving stem cell function.

There are several beneficial changes in your lifestyle that will help keep the stem cells functioning normally. The first thing you must do is stop smoking. It's a fact that smokers have decreased numbers of circulating stem cells; the more smoking, the lower the number of stem cells. Many health benefits occur when you quit smoking, but perhaps the most important benefit is that circulating stem cells increase in the blood within two weeks of quitting. Metabolic syndrome (and the associated inflammation and oxidation) is a real stem cell killer, so all the resulting tissue damage is compounded by a lack of stem cells.

Prevention of metabolic syndrome through good lifestyle and diet is essential to maintain healthy stem cells. Regular exercise not only improves your blood pressure and heart function, but it will also increase the number of circulating stem cells. The way to be kind to your stem cells is to lose weight, exercise, and eat a diet high in fruits, vegetables, good fats, and watch the glycemic index of the foods you eat. I'll discuss healthy diets later in the book, for now let's review some of the healthy foods that have been shown to improve stem cell numbers and function.

Spirulina (blue green algae):

Spirulina is a group of simple plant-like organisms, related to cyanobacterium, which are found in salt water and some large fresh water lakes. Spirulina is known as a potent antioxidant and anti-inflammatory nutrient source. Perhaps more important, however, is its effect on stem cells. When added to cultures of stem cells, spirulina helps to promote their growth. Preserving stem cell function is one of the main benefits of spirulina as demonstrated in the following study.

Severe inflammation, produced by an injection of lipopolysaccharide (LPS), causes a decrease in the number of stem cells in the brain. Researchers in Canada demonstrated how protective spirolina can be in this situation. They studied inflammation's effect on stems cells of rats. For twenty-eight days, one group was fed a regular diet, while the other group was fed a diet supplemented with spirulina. At the end of the diet period, the rats were given an infusion of LPS which causes a systemic inflammatory reaction similar to septic shock in humans. The rats fed spirulina were protected from the effects of the inflammation. Their brain tissue did not develop any decrease in the numbers of stem cells in comparison to the rats fed a regular diet. Without the protection of spirulina, systemic inflammation caused a decrease in stem cell number and damaged nerve cells resulted.

NT-020/ NutraStem®:

Other nutrients that help to enhance stem cell numbers and function include blueberries, green tea catechins, carnosine, and vitamin D. As all of these nutrients help to promote stem cell growth, they were combined and studied in combination. The resulting agent is called NT-020. Initial studies demonstrated that NT-020 effectively promoted the proliferation and growth of stem cells alone or in combination with other nutrients such as blue green algae, cacao and red sage. This turns out to be an important effect. As we age, inflammation damages our stem cells, decreasing their numbers and function. NT-020 has been found to decrease inflammation and increase the growth of stem cells in aging rats. NT-020, like spirulina, also protects stem cells from the effects of an infusion of LPS.

Stroke is a very serious and debilitating event that interrupts the blood supply and damages normal brain tissue including the brain's stem cells. Remember that stem cells are necessary for repair of damaged tissue, meaning the damage from a stroke is worse if the stem cells are not functioning properly. When used in an ischemic stroke model, NT-020 not only reduced the damage caused by the stroke, but also improved healing. Similar results were found when rats were supplemented with cacao and red sage, as long as the nutrients were supplemented *before* the stroke, not afterwards.

There are some impressive results with NT-020. It improves stem cell health and numbers and protects stem cells from insults like inflammation or stroke. NT-020 is available under the name NutraStem® and is marketed as natural support for your stem cells.

Folic acid:

Folic acid, also known as vitamin B-9, is necessary for the production of DNA, RNA, and for DNA repair. Normal cell growth and development depend on folic acid. Deficiencies of folic acid during pregnancy can lead to spina bifida, a condition in which the spinal cord does not form correctly. Sometimes, in severe cases, the brain does not form at all, which is known as anencephaly. Low folic acid levels can also cause damage to nerve tissues and stem cells. In mild cases, this can lead to numbness and tingling in the fingers and toes; in severe cases depression, dementia or seizures may result. Folic acid is a vitally important vitamin for the nervous system. Stem cells also rely on folic acid for proper function. Deficiency leads to death of stem cells in the nervous system, while supplementation improves growth and proliferation of nervous system stem cells.

Red Wine:

Red wine's many health benefits are all attributed to the polyphenol resveratrol, which has anti-oxidant properties, anti-aging benefits, and helps the heart and blood vessels. Resveratrol increases the growth and reproduction of stem cells in the blood of animals. This effect is taken advantage of in stem cell research. Scientists have been looking for a way to infuse stem cells to repair the damaged muscle from heart attacks. When resveratrol is added to stem cells, the life span of the stem cells is improved. These augmented stem cells are more effective at repairing damaged heart muscle after a heart attack.

If red wine helps stem cells, could any alcoholic beverage do the same? This is an interesting question and it was studied in Japan. Young volunteers were randomized to drink water, red wine, beer, or vodka daily for three weeks. Their blood was then assessed for circulating stem cells and stem cell function. After the three week test, only the red wine group was found to have a beneficial effect on the number of circulating stem cells, and stem cell function. It would seem that the resveratrol contained in wine, not alcohol, was responsible for the benefit. You can get this benefit from grapes or red wine; your choice.

There are two other commercially available supplements that have been shown to increase the numbers of circulating stem cells in your blood. They are Stem Enhance® and Stem Kine™. Stem Enhance® contains Aphanizomenon Flos-aquae and Mobilin, an L-selectin blocker which helps to release stem cells. Aphanizomenon is a type of cyanobacteria like spirulina. In a clinical study of normal volunteers, Stem Enhance® increased circulating stem cells by 25%. Stem Kine™ contains Ellagic acid, an anti-oxidant polyphenol, vitamin D, beta-glucan, and Lactobacillus bacteria. When given to healthy volunteers for 14 days, Stem Kine™ increased the percentage of circulating stem cells. Both of these products are able to increase circulating stem cells in healthy subjects, although studies in patients with disease have not been performed at this time.

In summary, stem cells are present at the beginning of life. They are cells with the potential to become any tissue, but their role later in life is to repair or replace damaged tissues. Poor lifestyle choices that lead to metabolic syndrome, diabetes, and high blood pressure will cause oxidation and inflammation which damages stem cells and causes premature aging. Good lifestyle choices will protect stem cells throughout your life. Additional supplements like blueberries, green tea, carnosine, vitamin D3 (Nutra-Stem®), spirulina, folic acid, cacao and red sage, red wine, Stem Enhance® and Stem Kine™ have been found to improve stem cell function.

IMMUNE SYSTEM:

The immune system is necessary for survival. It protects us against foreign invasion of bacteria, viruses, fungus, parasites and even cancer cells. These invaders can cause a lot of damage. The immune system is necessary to rid our bodies of infections and then allow the stem cells to repair or replace the damaged tissues. The immune system is composed of many parts that help to identify and tag invaders, kill the offending cell, and dispose of it. Don't forget, stem cells are important for producing cells of the immune system and so functioning stem cells are necessary for a strong immune system. What are the parts of the immune system?

The immune system is composed of cells, small proteins called immunoglobulins and attack complexes called complement. This system has two purposes; first and foremost, it determines self from non-self. The immune system determines which cells are supposed to be in our bodies and which are foreign. It determines this by recognizing small markers on our cells. Each person has a specific code on their cells that the immune system is familiar with. Any cell with that code is left alone, but if the code is not present on a cell, the cell is tagged with an immunoglobulin protein. Once tagged, an antigen-presenting cell attaches to it and presents it to an immune cell that will kill the foreign cell. The immunoglobulin proteins are specially made to react with only one type of cell. When you get an immunization shot, your body creates an immunoglobulin against that particular bacteria or virus in the shot. For example, a flu shot will produce immunoglobulins that will only recognize flu viruses, not bacteria. Your body is filled with thousands of varieties of immunoglobulins each programmed to recognize one particular infection.

Sometimes this system can be problematic, especially when someone needs a blood transfusion or an organ donation. In a blood transfusion, the body will not accept blood cells that are of a different blood type, and the ensuing conflict can sometimes be life-threating for the recipient of the transfusion. Organ transplants are more complicated. Organs cannot be matched perfectly unless the donated organ is from an identical twin. Strong immune suppressing drugs must be given to prevent rejection of the transplant.

The immune system is also able in some cases to detect cancer cells and destroy them. Since cancer cells are part of our body, most of the time they escape detection. Kidney cancers and melanomas however are vulnerable to the immune system. Therapies for these cancers try to harness the immune system to kill the cancer. Sometimes the tumor will completely melt away if the patient's own immune system can be harnessed to attack it.

Which organs make up the immune system?

Many organs in the body are part of the immune system: the tonsils, lymph nodes, thymus, spleen, appendix, Peyer's patches in the colon, and bone marrow. Bone marrow is the soft tissue on the inside of bones and it is the place in the body where blood cells are made. The bone marrow produces all the white blood cells, neutrophils, monocytes, and lymphocytes all of which are immune cells and help fight infections. The thymus is an organ that lies behind the breastbone. It is the place where T-cell lymphocytes mature. The spleen is located in the upper left side of your abdomen. It acts as a filter for the blood, filtering out old cells and bacteria. There are many immune cells in the spleen to fight infections of the blood. The colon lining contains islands of immune cells called Peyer's patches. The Peyer's patches in the gut are the first line of defense for bacteria in your food and they make up the largest immune organ in your body. Considering all the bacteria we eat each day, the gut immune system is doing a wonderful job. Lymph nodes and tonsils are part of the lymphatic system. These are small nodules attached to the lymph system that contain lymphocytes. They detect bacteria or viruses and destroy them. In the process, the lymph node can swell and become large and sometimes tender. This is why when you have a sore throat, your glands swell up.

The combination of immune cells and immunoglobulins form the backbone of the immune system. Other important parts include natural killer cells, which can kill bacteria without the rest of the immune system, phagocytic cells, which ingest bacteria and viruses, and the complement system, which helps the immune system destroy cells.

Immune system function can be evaluated in a number of ways. The three most basic tests are the total number of white blood cells, type of white blood cells and the levels of immunoglobulins. These tests can be drawn in any physician's office and these levels are often measured when an immune dysfunction is suspected. In some cases, the complement level can be assessed. More specialized testing, done in research institutions, includes measuring natural killer cell number and function. Studies of immune function and nutrition will often examine natural killer cells.

The immune system can be suppressed in many ways, making a person susceptible to infection. Many diseases, including autoimmune diseases (like rheumatoid arthritis and lupus), diabetes, anorexia nervosa, alcoholism, kidney diseases, lung disease, cancers and deficiencies of micronutrients like vitamin B-12, can lead to a poorly functioning immune system. Medicines such as the anti-inflammatory steroid prednisone, chemotherapy drugs, and drugs for organ transplant also suppress the immune system. People on these medicines need to be very careful about their increased risk of infection. Nutritional status also affects the immune system.

MALNUTRITION AND THE IMMUNE SYSTEM:

Malnutrition is the most common cause of immune deficiency in the world. An estimated 850 million people worldwide are malnourished. Malnutrition is one of the most important causes of infectious disease in developing countries and is responsible for approximately 300,000 deaths every year, including 50% of the deaths in children under the age of five. Malnutrition will affect the immune system in two ways, Protein-Energy Malnutrition (PEM) and micronutrient deficiency.

Protein-Energy-Malnutrition (PEM) occurs when the protein, carbohydrates and fat in the diet are not sufficient to meet the body's energy requirements. This causes muscle and fat wasting and decreased production of proteins, which are needed for immunoglobulins and the immune system. There is also a decreased production of white blood cells, specifically lymphocytes. People suffering from PEM typically develop respiratory infections, diarrheal illnesses, viral illnesses, bacterial illnesses, and atypical infections like fungus and tuberculosis. This type of malnutrition is most common in poverty-stricken areas of developing countries but it is also seen in the United States. Twenty-five percent of hospitalized pediatric patients in the United States, suffer from PEM while 55% of hospitalized adults and 85% of institutionalized adults suffer from malnutrition. It is incredible to think that severe malnutrition is common in hospitalized patients in the United States.

PEM is not the only malnutrition challenge facing us. Deficiencies of micronutrients are extremely common in the U.S. Micronutrients include vitamins, minerals, and dietary phytochemicals which we get from our diet. The best source of micronutrients is fruits and vegetables; you won't get the vast amounts of these in a vitamin pill. Micronutrients have important roles in immune cell functions and PEM generally also involves micronutrient deficiency. Isolated deficiencies are rare; except for vitamin A, iron, zinc, and vitamin D. Most malnourished people are deficient in multiple nutrients. The majority of people in the United States are deficient in micronutrients, because studies show that only 25% of Americans eat 5 or more servings of fruits and vegetables each day. The problem is junk food, fast food, processed foods, and comfort foods have little or no nutritional value. It is no wonder we have so many illnesses in this country with the way people eat. Why do you think you get so many colds or the flu every year? Could it be that your immune system is not working because you didn't feed it any micronutrients? This is why fruits and vegetables are so important.

Vitamin A Deficiency:

Vitamin A deficiency is a common cause of preventable blindness in the world. It is also a risk factor for infections and increased mortality. Severe deficiencies affect the immune system and account for an estimated 630,000 deaths from infection every year. A large percentage of deaths due to diarrhea, malaria and measles are attributed to vitamin A deficiency. Night blindness is one of the first symptoms of vitamin A deficiency. People become deficient in vitamin A when the diet lacks vegetables that contain carotenoids, animal meats, and fat. Fat helps us to absorb carotenes. Dietary sources of vitamin A include liver, milk, eggs, dark green leafy vegetables, yellow and orange non-citrus fruits (mangoes, apricots, and papayas), carrots, squash, and pumpkins.

Iron Deficiency:

Iron deficiency affects more than 2 billion people, mostly women and small children. Iron is an important component of hemoglobin found in red blood cells. Hemoglobin is necessary for transport of oxygen to the tissues. Iron is also necessary for growth and regulation of cells. Deficiency of iron can occur when there is inadequate intake during periods of rapid growth such as childhood, puberty, or pregnancy. Another cause in adults is blood loss through menstruation, parasite infections of the gut or other diseases of the bowel such as ulcers or cancer. Deficiency can cause damage to the nervous system and impairment of the immune system. Iron deficiency is an underlying factor in over 800,000 deaths each year. Iron is present in all plant foods, but is more plentiful and absorbable from meat. The body regulates absorption of iron so that under normal conditions you cannot absorb too much.

Zinc Deficiency:

Zinc is a mineral that is present throughout the body. It is necessary for the production of proteins and for cellular growth and differentiation. The best sources of zinc are oysters and shellfish. Deficiency usually occurs from inadequate intake, but phytic acid from nuts, seeds, and wheat bran inhibit zinc absorption, as well. Sometimes diarrheal illness will cause losses of zinc. Severe deficiency of zinc causes immune suppression, growth retardation, skin disorders, dysfunction of the testes, and bone marrow dysfunction. Mild deficiency increases the risk of infections like the common cold. Severe deficiency in developing countries is thought to be responsible for over 800,000 deaths annually.

Vitamin D deficiency:

Vitamin D is not a vitamin at all, but a secosteroid hormone that functions throughout the body. Deficiency of vitamin D causes bone disorders, immune dysfunction, autoimmune disease, heart disease, high blood pressure, and certain cancers. It is best known as a vitamin for bone health, but vitamin D receptors are present throughout the body and it is vital for a properly functioning immune system.[11] Vitamin D helps our immune system fight viral infections in your nose and other mucous membranes. Receptors in your nose recognize viruses and kill them on the spot, but they cannot function properly without vitamin D. Without vitamin D, we are susceptible to colds, flu and even tuberculosis. Studies in the United States show that the majority of Americans are deficient in vitamin D. This is because most

---

[11] Vitamin D helps by improving the barrier function in the upper airways which is very important during the cold and flu season. It tightens the gaps between cells and improves cell to cell communication. It also improves the function of Toll-like receptors (TLR). These receptors are present in the mucosal membranes of the nose and they function by detecting portions of cell membranes present on bacteria or viruses and then producing cathelicidin to kill the invading bug. Vitamin D works to prime the system thus making it more responsive to bacterial invasion. The TLR are the first line of defense against tuberculosis. Vitamin D, which is produced from sun exposure, helps fight tuberculosis. This is why patients in tuberculosis sanitariums were put in the sun as part of their treatment. We now have antibiotics to treat tuberculosis, but vitamin D is just as important today as in the past. Finally, vitamin D helps augment or prime the immune system to work better by improving the recruitment of immune cells.

of us spend our days indoors. The primary source for vitamin D is the sun and you won't get vitamin D under a fluorescent light or even sunlight through a window. It does not take long to get the vitamin D you need. Depending on your skin tone, 15 minutes might be enough to give you 15,000 units of vitamin D. Those persons with darker skin will need longer exposures since darker skin prevents the production of vitamin D. The best food sources of vitamin D are fatty fish, salmon, tuna, and cod, but you can also get vitamin D from fortified dairy products.

FOODS THAT BOOST YOUR IMMUNE SYSTEM:

There are many foods that have been found to improve immune function. Here are some of the best of those foods.

Garlic:

Garlic has been shown to stimulate immune cells including lymphocytes, macrophages, and natural killer cell activity. It primes these cells to be ready to rapidly fight infections and cancer cells.

Mushrooms:

Mushrooms have been a useful part of traditional Chinese medicine for centuries because they improve immune function. Thanks to their beta-glucan content, and polysaccharides that interact with the complement system, they enhance the maturation of antigen presenting cells in the bone marrow, and activate immune system cells including lymphocytes, macrophages, and natural killer cells. Mushrooms also help to modulate the immune system and, in autoimmune disease cases, can suppress the overactive immune system. Beta-glucans can inhibit the formation of cancer cells and stop cancer cells from growing. When given with chemotherapy or radiotherapy in mice, beta-glucans improve the recovery of white blood cells.

Fish Oil:

Fish oil is an omega-3 fatty acid composed of eisosapentanoic acid (EPA) and doxosopentanoic acid (DHA). Fatty fish was at one time thought to be unhealthy because of the fat content. Then studies of the Mediterranean diet, which is high in fish content, found fatty fish to be heart-healthful. Fish oil supplements have been found to be effective at lowering triglyceride levels in your blood and reducing the risk of heart attacks. There is a FDA approved fish oil supplement called Lovaza® which has been shown to drop triglyceride levels by 45%. It is available by prescription or in an over-the-counter version. There are data that fish oil will help reduce the risk of heart attack, and it is possibly effective at treating high blood pressure, rheumatoid arthritis, ADHD, depression or other mood disorders. Fish oil, when used as a supplement in baby formula, has been found to help the immune system develop faster. The EPA in fish oil has anti-inflammatory properties by preventing an overactive immune system. This is important: when the immune system runs out of control, we get chronic inflammation that can lead to many diseases.

Fish that are especially high in omega-3 fatty acids include mackerel, tuna, salmon, sturgeon, mullet, bluefish, anchovy, sardines, herring, trout, and menhaden. Fish oil supplements are usually made from mackerel, herring, tuna, halibut, salmon, and cod liver.

Glutamine:

Glutamine is an amino acid that is a building block for proteins and a fuel source for rapidly growing cells. Our bodies make glutamine and it is stored in the muscles and is rapidly released when it is needed. Body builders often use glutamine as a bulking agent because it serves as a building block for proteins. It is also an important part of the immune system. The gut is loaded with immune cells (lymphocytes) which are located in Peyer's patches. Under stress conditions, like severe infections, surgery, or cancer, the body depletes glutamine rapidly. Without this food source, the immune system, and tissue repair are impaired. It is beneficial to supplement glutamine during these times of stress.

Glutamine has been shown to decrease the infection rate in severely ill patients in hospitals through its effects on lymphocytes and the gut. In cancer patients, glutamine can help prevent sores in the mouth or diarrhea caused from chemotherapy, and nerve pain from paclitaxel. Glutamine can also help people with cancer or AIDS gain weight.

Chinese Herbs:

Herbs have been a part of traditional Chinese medicine for centuries. Their beneficial effects come from the polyphenols and saponins they contain. Herbs are used for a variety of conditions because they decrease inflammation and improve the immune system.

Chinese herbs that have beneficial effects on the immune system include Astragalus mongholicus, Acanthopanux senticosus, Panax notoginseng, Tripterygium wilfordii, Aconitum, and Artemesiae. Astragalus in particular has been found to restore the immune system function. Astragalus helps activate T-cell lymphocytes after chemotherapy.

Probiotics:

Probiotics are bacteria that are necessary for normal function of the gut and immune system. The large intestines are colonized with bacteria early during fetal development. After birth, the gut is colonized with bifidobacteria especially if the infant is breast-fed. These bacteria have several purposes. They help to modulate gene expression in the intestines and set up normal colonization of beneficial bacteria. They prevent infectious diarrhea by preventing the growth of harmful bacteria. They influence the motility and blood flow to the intestines. They also stimulate the immune system and thus prevent transfer of bacteria from the intestines to the blood system. In a malnutrition model in mice, fermented milk with probiotic bacteria helped restore normal immune function quicker than a normal diet did. Probiotics are also effective at resolving infectious diarrhea, especially antibiotic associated diarrhea due to Clostridium dificile.

Micronutrients:

Micronutrients are vitamins, minerals, and phytonutrients found in small amounts in the foods we eat, especially fruits and vegetables. Several studies on malnutrition have now been completed that demonstrate that supplementation can improve immune function. The most beneficial supplements appear to be zinc, vitamins E, A, C and beta-carotene. Dr. R.K. Chandra studied the immune system effects of a multivitamin supplement containing retinol, beta-carotene, thiamine, riboflavin, niacin, pyridoxine, folate, B12, vitamin C, vitamin D, vitamin E, iron, copper, selenium, iodine, calcium, and magnesium. In elderly patients, this multi-nutrient supplement did improve immune function after 12 months. Some studies suggest an improvement with zinc or vitamin E supplements. Caution is advised in taking mega-doses of any synthetic vitamin. They all have associated side effects that are more common at higher doses. Natural whole food sources are always the best source of micronutrients. A natural whole food supplement called Juice Plus+® has also been shown to improve immune function and decrease the symptoms of the cold virus. Since most of us don't eat enough fruits and vegetables I would recommend whole food sources of nutrition like juicing or the whole food supplement Juice Plus+® to supplement your diet.

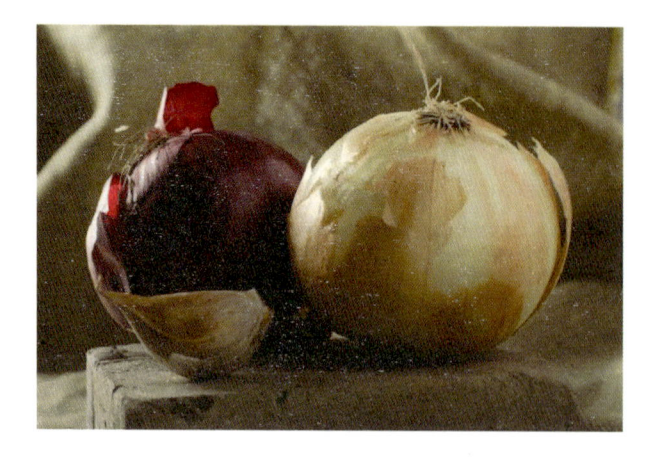

3. HOW TO TAKE CHARGE OF YOUR HEALTH THROUGH DIET

Modern medicine has reached great heights of sophistication and ability. Unfortunately, a negative side effect of the powers of modern medicine is that we now trust our doctors' ability to treat any illness too much and we take little responsibility for our own health. We don't put much thought or energy into the daily work of healthful living and, as I will show, this can have some serious health consequences.

We are continuously bombarded by advertisements in print, on billboards, the radio and television that promise to meet the human desires for happiness and self-worth through food, fashion, and makeup. Food commercials, in particular, dazzle our eyes with colors and textures in an attempt to compel us to buy a certain product. No one likes the feeling of hunger, so we are encouraged to eat often to be satisfied and happy. Those enticing advertisements tell us of the wide array of things we could eat without telling us what we should eat.

Have you ever stopped to think how has the human diet changed since the beginning of time? Not many people are aware of how much our foods have changed. This is an important idea because changes in the human diet are directly responsible for the increase in obesity and chronic diseases we now experience.

Early human ancestors were present on earth two million years ago. These nomadic peoples lived near the equator in small groups. Scientists have determined what a typical diet would be for humans living two million years ago. They hunted wild animals and ate whatever plant foods they could find. There was no organized farming or domesticated animals, so they are called hunter-gatherers. The hunter-gatherer, or Paleolithic diet, was quite different from our modern diet. It consisted of wild meat, seafood, vegetables, nuts and berries.

The world changed approximately 10,000 years ago when a new era began: the Neolithic time period. During this time, the last ice age passed and the planet became more hospitable to humans. As humans increased in numbers, they began to migrate north and south away from the equator. As populations grew and spread over the globe, the nomadic hunter-gatherer lifestyle was abandoned. Organized populations developed an agricultural based diet and they domesticated animals for protein. During the Neolithic period, humans learned to use grains such as barley and wheat, and oils such as olive oil. They consumed dairy products, made wine and beer, and used salt as a preservative. These changes were gradual and there was much variation in what populations ate based on their location. Diets in extreme northern climates included more fish and less vegetation because of the short growing season, while more temperate areas could incorporate more farmed fruits and vegetables. Olive oil was present in the Mediterranean areas. The development of trade routes made it possible to transport exotic foods to other areas of the world. Diets during the Neolithic age remained relatively unchanged for thousands of years, but in the last century food around the world changed radically.

Since the Industrial Age, the human lifestyle changed considerably as communication developed. First, distant societies were connected by roads and railways, then the telegraph, then the telephone, satellite, and now the internet. We are connected to other people like never before in human history, and our diet and food supply has changed to meet our needs. Meals can be prepared quickly and mechanically, purchased ready-made or at a restaurant. Technologies over the last 120 years have been developed to enhance not only the appeal of food but also the shelf life. The hunter-gatherer period lasted 2 million years, the Neolithic period 10,000 years, and modern processed foods 120 years. It is during this last time period that we have seen the introduction of Coca Cola® (1886), Cracker Jack® (1893), Jell-O® (1897), Corn Flakes® (1900), Oreo® cookies (1912), Marshmallow Fluff® (1920), Kool Aid® (1920), Velveeta® cheese food (1928), Twinkies® (1930), Lay's® potato chips (1932), and Skippy® peanut butter (1932). This is a diverse group of foods, all delicious tasting, and they have three things in common; sugar, fat, and salt.

Sugars, fats, and salts have always been present in our diets. During the hunter-gatherer and Neolithic periods, our diets contained fats present in meats, nuts and later as processed oils like olive oil, sugars in fruits, complex carbohydrates in grains and nuts, and very little salt. The major change in diet during the last 100 years has been that sugars, fats, and salt are now added to foods to enhance the flavor. Foods are commonly fried in oil and contain added sugar and salt. The salt and sugar add taste and the fat adds texture and enhances the favorability of the sugar and salt. A combination of all three, a terrible tantalizing trio, make food very tasty and, as we shall see, difficult to resist.

The trio of sugar, fat and salt creates health problems that affect individuals and impact society as a whole. Bad fats increase inflammation and oxidation. Sugar causes increased weight and inflammation, oxidation, diabetes, heart disease and cancer. Salt leads to high blood pressure and some forms of cancer. Just how much more fat, sugar and salt are we eating these days? Let's find out.

Sugar, although introduced thousands of years ago, was very expensive and only consumed by the very wealthy. In 1900, Americans ate an average of one pound of sugar each year. Now, with modern processing, inexpensive sugar or syrups are easily added to foods so we eat an average of one hundred and eighty two pounds a year – each! How is that possible? A twelve-ounce soda contains 10 teaspoons of sugar, three sodas contain ¼ pound of sugar. Factor in the other added sugars in drinks and foods, and the amount escalates to ½ pound or more of sugar a day. On average, Americans eat 53 teaspoons of sugar a day. From 1 pound of sugar a year to 182 pounds, the cause of the American epidemic of obesity and diabetes is quite clear, isn't it?

A healthy diet should contain no more than 20% of its calories from fat. Americans eat 65 pounds of fat each year, which is 50% more than we consumed in 1950. We consume 2/3 of this fat in the form of salad oils, cooking oils, and fried foods. Beyond the increase in calories, there are obvious health implications of eating this much fat. High fat diets, especially saturated fats cause your blood vessels to clamp down and the effect lasts for hours. This is one reason heart attacks can occur after a large fatty meal. Polyunsaturated omega-6 fats, like those found in animal fats and corn oil, increase inflammation and oxidation which cause chronic diseases like atherosclerosis, heart disease, stroke and cancer. The good news is, monounsaturated fats like olive oil and fish oil are safer and do not cause chronic diseases or inflammation.

Sodium Chloride otherwise known as table salt has been used for thousands of years as a preservative to prevent spoilage. Until the invention of modern refrigeration, salt was regularly used to preserve meat, and is still valuable in curing bacon, ham, or other meat, and can be used in pickling vegetables. A teaspoon of salt contains approximately 2,400mg of sodium and the recommended daily allowance of sodium is 1,500 mg a day. The minimum amount needed to live is 180-500 mg but Americans eat up to 3,500 mg a day. Most of that salt is found in processed foods. Nine out of ten Americans eat too much salt, which causes high blood pressure, heart failure, and some forms of cancer. You may not be adding salt, but unfortunately with processed food, the salt has already been added. You need to read nutrition labels to find out how much sodium you are eating each day.

Why do Americans like to eat so much sugar, salt and fat? These ingredients not only taste good, they are addictive. The answer to why we eat so much can be found in our brains. Research has demonstrated that these three flavors will actually lead to release of various powerful chemicals that affect your brain. The response to eating processed foods high in fat, sugar and salt is the release of endorphins and dopamine. The endorphins have an effect similar to morphine, producing pleasure. The dopamine is a chemical associated with movement, memory, attention and problem solving. When these two chemicals are stimulated it not only produces pleasure but the motivation to seek out more of the same food. This combination is similar for any addictive substance and addictive behaviors have been demonstrated in animals and humans. Rats will wander through mazes, climb steep walls, and even cross an electrified floor to get to junk food. Studies in humans demonstrate if a free vending machine is available, people will visit it repeatedly until they have unthinkingly added several thousand extra calories a day to their caloric intake.

Food researchers and marketers know how appealing these flavors are to people. They carefully develop their recipes and then confirm the results with taste tests. The end result is a tasty food that people love to eat. The problem is processed foods have too much sugar, fat and salt and not enough nutrition. In other words, processed foods contain empty calories. This is the reason adults weigh on average 10 pounds more today than in 1960 and the obesity rate has increased 50% since 1990.

With increasing weight, naturally, comes the desire to lose it. The weight loss industry has taken notice of people's desire to lose weight. The ever-growing weight loss industry includes diet plans like Jenny Craig and Weight Watchers®, plans that prepare and deliver meals to your door, and quick weight loss fad diets.

The surgical community has even joined in, as cosmetic surgeons routinely remove fat surgically. Bariatric surgeons alter the stomach through bypass surgery or lap band procedures to induce weight loss. Unfortunately, surgical procedures can be associated with complications. Many diet plans are no more than a quick fix promising weight loss in a few weeks with no plan to maintain the lost weight, and some diets are so restrictive that in the long run, they would cause nutritional deficiencies of key vitamins. It is more harmful to repeatedly lose and gain weight than to maintain a healthy, nutrient-filled diet and maintain the same weight.

There are three essential attributes of any weight loss plan: It helps you safely lose weight, it contains all the necessary nutrients for health, and it is a meal plan that you can remain on and maintain your weight and health. If your weight loss plan doesn't meet these criteria, drop it. It is not good for you.

LOSE WEIGHT FAST:

The diet faddism in America.

There are so many diets out there it boggles the mind. A quick search on the internet reveals there are approximately 62,000 books about dieting for sale. The promises are many and varied: one diet is for busy women, no starving, no restrictions, no workouts; others promise weight loss in sixty days, or fourteen days, or even one week.

Each one seems better than the last. Diets take many forms: low-carb, low-fat, liquid diets, grapefruit diets, detox diets, cabbage soup diets, macrobiotic diets, juice diet, and even a lemon and cayenne pepper diet. The problem with fad diets is they don't work for long because the more restrictive a diet is, the less likely that diet will be followed long term.

The best method of dieting is to pick healthful foods and maintain a healthy portion of calories. Let's look at a handful of diets and weight loss plans that have been scientifically studied and examine them as lifestyle plans, as our ultimate goal is to be healthy and free from disease. It would be impossible to discuss all of the thousands of diets in the world, and I also do not mean to exclude any other good diets. Many good diets have not been studied scientifically. I selected these diets based on research that is available in the medical literature. We'll discuss the Paleolithic (or hunter-gatherer) diet, low carbohydrate/Atkins diet, DASH diet, Mediterranean diet, and vegetarian/vegan diets. It is very important that you study each diet to decide which is best for you. They all have strong points, but no one diet suits all people. Remember, the ultimate goal is to get the right nutrition to prevent oxidation, inflammation, metabolic syndrome, diabetes, heart disease, and cancer, and to ensure your genes, DNA, immune system and stem cells are in good working order.

PALEOLITHIC DIET/ HUNTER-GATHERER DIET

Humans have evolved and changed over millions of years. Current data shows that we were hunter-gatherers from 2.6 million to approximately 10,000 years ago. Although our lifestyle has changed tremendously in the last 10,000 years, our DNA and genes have not. Supporters of the Paleolithic diet say modern diseases are due to a lifestyle for which our bodies were not designed. Our ancestors did not eat processed foods, trans fats, sugar or salt. The Paleo diet's supporters maintain that diseases like high blood pressure, diabetes, heart disease and cancer did not exist until humans left the hunter-gatherer diet and lifestyle.

It is not possible to know exactly how the daily diet of the Paleolithic human, of course. The foods these nomads ate were based on what foods were available at the time, a menu that would have been affected by the season of the year and weather conditions. One thing is clear: our ancestors were not vegetarians like apes and monkeys. Animal based protein was essential in the development of our complex brains. Our ancestors ate a diet of lean meat, vegetables, fruits and nuts. The amount of meat varied on tribe and was as little as 30% or as high as 80% of their diet. Modern hunter-gatherer societies will eat a diet of 45-65% animal meat. It is somewhat astounding, but they also don't suffer from many of the chronic diseases that plague us. So is this the best diet for you? Let's look at some of the studies.

A look at modern hunter-gatherer societies confirms that they consume more than the recommended portions of meat and fat than current guidelines in the United States, but have low cholesterol levels and low rates of heart disease. It may seem counterintuitive, but a high meat hunter-gatherer diet does not cause heart disease. The key is the meat is lean and wild, not domesticated and corn-fed and there is no sugar or processed foods.

In Australia, diabetic Aborigines were returned to their historic hunter-gatherer lifestyle to see if this affected their health. After only 7 weeks of a hunter-gatherer diet of meat, vegetables and nuts, they lost on average 17 pounds and more importantly, their diabetes either went away or markedly improved.

Studies are demonstrating how this diet of lean meat, fruits and vegetables is also healthy for non-hunter-gatherers. The Paleolithic diet is an effective way to lose weight in overweight individuals. Healthy overweight volunteers lost an average of 5 pounds after only 3 weeks on a hunter-gatherer diet. In studies from Europe, the Paleolithic diet has been shown to improve blood pressure, drop blood sugar, insulin and cholesterol levels in healthy volunteers after only 7 days.

A hunter-gatherer diet is certainly a diet to consider. Multiple studies have shown that a diet of lean meat, fruits, vegetables and nuts that excludes grains, dairy and legumes is very healthy. It has also been shown to reverse diabetes and heart disease in individuals from modern society. This diet consistently leads to weight loss, improved blood sugars and insulin levels, and even compares favorably to a Mediterranean style diet in health benefits. It seems especially suited for cardiovascular health and diabetes. From this high meat diet we move to look at another high meat, high fat, and low carbohydrate diet: the Atkins diet.

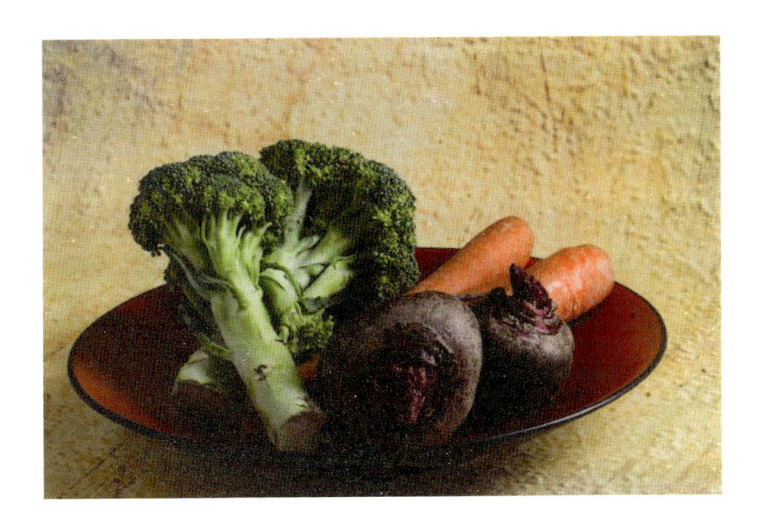

Dr. Bob Avery MD, FACP

LOW CARBOHYDRATE, ATKIN'S TYPE DIET

When he published his first book in the 1970's, Dr. Robert Atkins set off a revolution in eating. His legacy has continued with his second book published in 2002 and continues even after his death in 2003. In 1970, a low fat, high carbohydrate diet was thought to be the best way to lose weight. Fat contains many calories and was thought to be the cause of obesity and heart disease. Official dietary recommendations at that time consistently recommended a diet comprised of 20-30% fat, 30% protein and 40-50% carbohydrates. The old food pyramid reflected these recommendations. Dr. Atkins turned the dietary world on its head with his revolutionary concept that carbohydrates, not fat, cause weight gain.

The basic concept of the Atkins diet is to change the way the body processes and stores energy. The basic energy source in our food is from carbohydrates including sugars, grains and starches. Through a series of chemical reactions, carbohydrates are converted to glucose for immediate use as energy, or converted to fat for storage. Blood sugar and insulin levels increase in response to the carbohydrates. The insulin drives the sugar into cells to use for energy or to be turned into fat for storage. The idea behind the Atkins is to limit carbohydrates and force the body to get energy from stored fat. Without excess carbohydrates no excess fat can be formed. This process causes the formation of ketones from fat to be used for energy and so is sometimes referred to a ketogenic diet. Over the last 40 years, many studies have shown that low carbohydrate diets are associated with a significant amount of weight loss, but there have been questions about this diet. Is it safe? Is it healthy?

There has been much controversy surrounding the Atkins diet. In his original concept, the meal plan included very low carbohydrates, but all the meat and fat you wanted. Atkins dieters do not count calories, only carbohydrates. Any source of meat or fat was allowed, including saturated fats. Since high saturated fat diets lead to heart disease, there was immediate criticism of the Atkins method. Critics claimed it would lead to heart disease, kidney stones, increase inflammation and the ketones would make the person feel sick. What about the effect on diabetes? A low carbohydrate diet should be beneficial. Well, we'll look at some of the most recent research about the Atkins diet. It is important to note the Atkins meal plan has actually been amended over the years. The current model places less emphasis on saturated fats and red meats and more on vegetables and some fruits.

There are 4 phases to the Atkins weight loss plan: induction, ongoing weight loss, pre-maintenance, and lifetime maintenance. The induction phase is the most extreme, allowing only 20 grams of net carbohydrates a day. In this phase the person will generally lose up to 15 pounds. Phase II allows slightly more carbohydrates, but dieters can expect to lose another 10 pounds or so. During phase III, dieters gradually increase the carbohydrates 10 grams a week until reaching the goal weight. At this point, dieters continue in a maintenance phase. Exercise is not discouraged, but dieters may be weakened because of the lack of carbohydrates and should take care to maintain safe activity levels during the initial phases of the diet.

A low carbohydrate diet has been found to consistently lead to weight loss, as much as 30 pounds in some studies. Waist size drops and there is an improvement in blood pressure. Laboratory tests show a drop in blood sugar and insulin level consistent with improvement of diabetes. Heart function improves and, in one study, exercise tolerance was not affected. Some studies have shown an improvement in cholesterol levels, while some studies show no change or only a slight increase. When compared to a standard low fat diet, many studies show equivalent results in the categories of weight loss and diabetes, but show improved cholesterol and blood vessel function in the Atkins dieters. The difference may lie in which fats are allowed in the diet. The original Atkins concept did not limit saturated fats, which have been associated with inflammation, oxidation, and heart disease. Newer versions of the diet encourage healthier fats and lean meats, resulting in an improved, healthier diet overall.

When a low carbohydrate diet limits saturated fats and instead focuses on healthier mono-unsaturated fats like fish oil and olive oil, beneficial effects on cholesterol level and blood vessel function result. One notable study from the United Arab Emirates showed benefits in weight, blood sugar, insulin, cholesterol levels, and inflammation with this type of diet. More recent studies on low carbohydrate diets report different results than the initial studies, due mainly to the change in fat content. Omega-3 fats like olive oil and fish oil are very healthy and make a low carbohydrate diet more heart friendly, but what about diabetes?

When the data from eighteen studies was combined to determine how fat and carbohydrates affect diabetes, the results were not surprising. A low carbohydrate, high fat diet was associated with improved markers of diabetes while the combined analysis confirmed that high carbohydrate diets worsen diabetes. The benefits were best if the fat content was mono-unsaturated fats. After two years on a low carbohydrate diet, the risk of heart disease drops.

DASH DIET

The DASH diet, or the Dietary Approaches to Stop Hypertension, is a diet scientifically developed to reduce weight and reduce high blood pressure. It has received high marks from multiple groups and was ranked #1 best, healthiest diet by *US News and World Reports* in November 2011. It is also endorsed by the National Heart Lung and Blood Institute, the American Heart Association, and the MAYO clinic. It is a 28 day meal plan that is set out and easy to follow. People on this diet may see their blood pressure drop in as little as 14 days, and if you remain on this diet long term, it has been found to decrease the risk of stroke, heart disease, kidney stones, and even some cancers.

The DASH diet was developed based on scientific studies that demonstrated lifestyle modifications could lower blood pressure. In fact, lifestyle modification is still considered the first step in treatment of early hypertension. The seventh report of the Joint National

Committee on the Prevention, Detection, Evaluation and Treatment of High Blood Pressure recommends weight loss, DASH diet, limiting sodium to 2.4 grams daily, moderate alcohol use, and exercise as an integral part in the management of high blood pressure. What is a DASH diet? The diet focuses on fruits, vegetables, low fat dairy products, poultry, fish, whole grains, nuts, but limited amounts of red meat, sweets, soft drinks, total and saturated fats. A sample of the DASH diet is shown in the following table.

Type of Food	Servings for 2000 Cal/day diet
Grains, at least 3 whole grains	7-8
Fruits	4-5
Vegetables	4-5
Low fat/non-fat Dairy	2-3
Fish, poultry, lean meats	2 or less
Nuts, seeds, legumes	4-5 weekly
Fats and sweets	limited

When compared to a typical American diet, the DASH diet will decrease blood pressure, especially when it incorporates low salt intake. Blood pressures drop on a DASH diet in both normal people and those with elevated blood pressure. Greater than 50% of the participants in

DASH diet studies were minorities and women, demonstrating that the diet will be beneficial to a wide variety of ethnic groups. African Americans are sensitive to salt, so the low-salt DASH diet is especially beneficial to this group. How well can it work? The combination of DASH diet and low salt can drop blood pressure by 11.5 points in people with high blood pressure. This is a similar drop seen with high blood pressure medicine. The amazing part is you can improve your blood pressure by diet alone in as little as thirty days without medicines.

Although weight loss is not the sole purpose of a DASH diet, studies have shown a modest decrease in weight in individuals who remain on the diet. One notable study of people with high blood pressure and metabolic syndrome compared the DASH alone or with the addition of a low sodium vegetable juice for 12 weeks. As expected, more than 50% of the individuals had normalization of their blood pressures, but after 12 weeks, those on the DASH diet and vegetable juice lost an average of 5 pounds.

When weight control is the goal, the benefits of the DASH are even better. In a study from Duke University called the ENCORE study, the DASH diet was compared to DASH plus weight management activities. The DASH diets were the same but the weight management group underwent behavioral sessions to develop proper eating, and they also had supervised exercise three times a week. Those in the weight management group lost an average of twenty pounds each, their blood pressure dropped further, and markers of heart function improved.

The benefits of the DASH diet pay off even more if the diet is followed for years. When populations of women on the diet are studied for many years, we find that those on a DASH-like diet have a 25% lower risk of heart disease, 20% lower risk of stroke, and a 37% decreased risk of heart failure compared to women who ate a typical diet.

Men and women who remain on a DASH diet will decrease their risk of kidney stones by 40-45%. The combination of decreased animal protein and increased fruits and vegetables was key to preventing kidney stones. Women who follow this diet will also decrease their risk of certain types of breast cancer by 20%. The DASH diet is one of the most thoroughly studied diets. It demonstrates the health benefits of fruits, vegetables, whole grains, nuts, and restriction of red meat, saturated and total fat. It was developed to treat high blood pressure, but as you can see, its benefits, which include decreased risk of heart disease, stroke, kidney stones, and breast cancer, demonstrate the power of a healthful diet.

MEDITERRANEAN DIET

A Mediterranean diet is based on the typical diet naturally occurring in the regions around the Mediterranean Sea and stretching in to the Middle East. It varies by regions but essentially is composed of fish or poultry as a protein source, some red meat, and fruits, vegetables, olives, beans, whole grains, some dairy, moderate amounts of red wine, and olive oil. Interest in this diet began fifty years ago when studies found that men on the Greek island of Crete had a very low risk of heart disease and certain cancers, in spite of their high fat diet. Another study of 22,000 Greeks demonstrated that stricter adherence to a Mediterranean style diet resulted in a 25% reduction in mortality over the 44 months of the study. Researchers began to take notice of the Mediterranean style diet that could prevent heart disease and lower mortality. The question for researchers was: why would this high fat diet be so beneficial for the heart?

There are many features about the Mediterranean diet that make it beneficial for the heart: fruits, vegetables, fish, and olive oil. Increasing your intake of fruits and vegetables improves risk factors of heart disease. Fish, on the other hand, is not just an alternate source of protein to red meat but it is also beneficial to the heart, and fatty fish, containing omega-3 fish oils, are particularly beneficial. Fish oils, when eaten in fish or as a capsule, have been found to lower triglyceride levels in the blood, lower heart rate, lower blood pressure, decrease inflammation, and improve the function of the blood vessels. Finally, some of the heart healthy benefits are due to a key component of the Mediterranean diet: olive oil. Olive oil, like fish oil, is an omega-3 fat, which has beneficial effects on blood lipids and the blood vessels, and has anti-oxidant and anti-inflammatory properties. It is the combination of fruits, vegetables, fish, and olive oil that make the Mediterranean diet so healthy.

When compared to a typical low-fat diet, a Mediterranean diet supplemented with olive oil or nuts is more effective at dropping blood pressure, blood sugar, cholesterol levels, and the inflammatory marker

C-reactive protein. Another study comparing low-fat diet to a low carbohydrate Mediterranean diet in diabetic dieters showed greater improvement in blood sugar levels and heart disease risk factors with the low-carbohydrate Mediterranean diet. One amazing study showed that after four years, people on the Mediterranean style diet were 40% less likely to require medications to control their diabetes.

The Mediterranean diet benefits also extend to those who have already had a heart attack. In Lyon, France, patients who had a heart attack were randomized to eat either a Mediterranean style diet or the American Heart Association Step I Diet. They were then observed for second heart events or death. The risk of a second heart attack was decreased 73% with the Mediterranean diet and the risk of dying within 27 months dropped by 70% compared to the AHA Step 1 Diet. This incredible benefit occurs because the Mediterranean diet improves oxidation and cardiovascular risk factors. If weight loss is the goal, then a low carbohydrate Mediterranean style diet can be used. Dropping the amount of carbohydrates will effectively produce weight loss while improving blood sugar and cholesterol levels.

Beyond heart health, the Mediterranean diet also has been found to decrease the risk of certain kinds of cancer. Observational studies of large populations in Europe and the United States have found a decreased risk of breast cancer, stomach cancer and prostate cancer in those who follow a Mediterranean style diet.

Since the optimum diet for weight loss has not been determined yet, the Dietary Intervention Randomized Controlled Trial compared three weight loss plans, low-fat restricted calorie diet (traditional American Heart Association), Mediterranean style restricted calorie diet, and a low-carbohydrate non-calorie restricted diet (based on Atkins diet). The results were mixed, and don't really determine a clear winner. Weight loss was greatest with the Mediterranean and low carbohydrate diets. Inflammation and lipids were improved the most with the low carbohydrate diet, while blood sugars in diabetics dropped the most on the Mediterranean diet. Longer follow up of 2 years showed continued health benefits of these diets but there was not one that was clearly superior to the others.

VEGETARIAN/VEGAN DIETS

Vegetarians do not eat meat, fish, or poultry and strict vegan diets also avoid dairy and eggs. There are some variations to these diets; some forms restrict even more foods. Sometimes people are vegetarian for religious reasons, sometimes out of personal preference. Vegetarians can be found in most countries and the largest vegetarian community is found in India, where 35% of the citizens are vegetarian. Some have been concerned that a vegetarian diet does not offer enough nutrition or protein to be healthy, but expert reviews by the American Dietetic Association and the Dieticians of Canada have determined that a well-planned vegetarian diet provides adequate nutrition for all stages of life.

Vegetarian diets are rich in carbohydrates, fiber, omega-6 fatty acids, carotenoids, folic acid, vitamin C, vitamin E, and magnesium. They are relatively low in protein, omega-3 fatty acids, retinol, vitamin B-12, zinc, and iron. Strict vegan dieters will have additional low intakes of vitamin D and calcium by excluding fish and dairy products. Finally, since the source of vitamin B-12 is dairy and eggs, there is a risk of vitamin B-12 deficiency as well. It is advisable that vegan vegetarians take a vitamin B-12 supplement.

The combination of vitamin D and calcium deficiencies in strict vegans are thought to increase the risk of osteoporosis, but osteoporosis and bone fractures in vegetarians are actually unusual. Studies comparing vegans to non-vegetarians found little or no difference in bone density. Bone fractures are also unusual as long as the intake of protein is adequate, because the risk of osteoporotic bone fractures is affected not only by calcium and vitamin D but also by protein intake. Only vegetarians with the lowest protein intake are at an increased risk of fractures. Adequate levels of vegetable proteins in the form of beans and nuts are easy enough to achieve and will reverse this risk.

The health benefits of a vegetarian style diet are many. Vegetarians and vegans typically weigh less, have lower cholesterol levels, lower blood pressure and reduced risk of heart disease, stroke and some forms of cancer, especially if they are avid eaters of nuts. Here are some recent research findings relating to these diets.

Compared directly to meat eaters, vegetarians have lower blood pressure and lower cholesterol and healthier blood vessels. The increased fiber in their diet also decreases the risk of diverticular disease. Diverticular disease is characterized by weakening of the bowel wall causing areas where the colon balloons out. These diverticula can be painful or become infected and sometimes that part of the colon needs to be removed surgically to treat the disease. In populations that eat a high fiber diet, diverticulosis is non-existent.

Vegetarian diets will also decrease the risk of diabetes because of weight loss and the anti-oxidant effects of fruits and vegetables. A vegetarian style diet has been found to be better than a standard diabetes diet at controlling blood sugar and lipid levels. Interestingly, a low carbohydrate, vegetarian diet has been developed. The so called "Eco Atkins" diet improves not only weight, but blood sugar, blood pressure, and cholesterol as well. Since vegetarian diets are so healthy, they have been proposed as one way to improve the childhood obesity problem in America. Can you imagine how healthy our country would be if our children started eating a healthy diet and continued into adulthood?

Do vegetarians live longer? Many people think so. Some experts suggest a high intake of meat is associated with chronic diseases and increased mortality, so it seems to be a reasonable thought that vegetarians would live longer. While it is true that vegetarians are generally healthier and live longer than unhealthy people, studies comparing vegetarians to health conscious individuals that exercise and do not smoke show no difference in how long they live. The key to a longer life is a healthful lifestyle. All of these diets are healthful. There is not one that is best for all. It is very important to pick a diet plan that you can follow for life.

SUPPLEMENTS

If everyone in America ate the healthiest foods, it would be unusual to see anyone with heart disease, high blood pressure, diabetes, cancer or chronic diseases. We have all the tools but we are not, in general, a healthy population. Americans simply do not eat the right foods. With all the information available about diets and what to eat, it would seem perfectly simple for everyone to pick a diet, follow a plan, and become healthy. However, according to the Centers for Disease Control and Prevention (CDC), only 25% of adults eat the recommended five or more servings of fruits and vegetables daily, and 40% eat two or fewer servings daily. How many servings of fruits and vegetables should one eat per day? The CDC recommends two cups of fruit and three cups of vegetables daily. The National Cancer Institute recommends five servings of fruits and vegetables daily to help prevent cancers. The American Institute for Cancer Research recommends eating more fruits, vegetables and healthy grains, but according to a WebMD article, "5-a-Day May Not be Enough", a study in Europe showed that only people who ate eight or more servings of fruits and vegetables on a daily basis decreased their risk of heart disease by 22%. Keep in mind that healthful diets like the hunter-gatherer, Mediterranean, DASH, and vegetarian include at least eight to ten servings of fruits and vegetables daily. Although the government recommends five servings a day, it is apparent that eating more servings is better for the body and necessary to prevent diseases and get you off medicines.

So how do we get the daily nutrition we need if we don't get enough fruits and vegetables? The most common way in the United States is to take vitamins. The use of vitamin supplements is on the rise in the United States. According to the CDC, 40% of Americans use vitamin supplements.

The problem with vitamin supplements is the lack of scientific evidence that they prevent any disease; therefore, they are misleading to consumers who look to supplements for nutrition. Official recommendations for vitamins reflect this concern. The CDC recommends getting important nutrients directly from fruits and vegetables. An official American Institute for Cancer Research (AICR) panel statement reported in 2008 that whole foods, not dietary supplements, play a role in preventing cancer. The American Heart Association recommends a diet rich in fruits and vegetables to help prevent heart disease, because there is insufficient data from studies that antioxidant vitamins prevent heart disease.

Antioxidant vitamins have not been found to help prevent heart failure, to halt progression of coronary disease, or diabetes. Multiple trials have also failed to show that vitamin E or selenium can prevent lung cancer or prostate cancer. One very concerning trial, the CARET trial, showed that beta-carotene supplementation in smokers increased the risk of lung cancer instead of preventing it. Other trials of vitamin A or its retinoid derivatives have not been shown to decrease the risk of lung cancer either, so it is increasingly clear that antioxidant vitamins will not prevent diseases.

The potential dangers of vitamins have also been examined. Certain vitamins like A, D, E, and K are stored in the body's fat and can accumulate to toxic levels if taken in excess. Vitamin A or retinoids can cause nausea, headaches, liver toxicity and even coma in high doses. Vitamin E in high doses can cause bleeding, blurred vision and headaches. Vitamin B-6 can cause numbness and tingling. Vitamin B-3 (niacin) can cause flushing, diarrhea, liver damage, and dry skin. Vitamin B-9 (folate) can cause nausea, abdominal pain, and rash. Vitamin C can cause flushing, nausea, headache, and increased oxalate in the urine. Vitamin D can cause nausea, constipation, sleepiness, and high calcium in the blood. As you can see, high doses of any vitamin are associated with many side effects. Analyses of multiple trials (otherwise known as a meta-analysis), suggests there may be an increased chance of death in those who take antioxidant vitamins. There is little evidence that vitamins prevent disease and they may even be harmful. Indiscriminant use in hopes of preventing disease is not recommended.

Vitamins do have a role for certain people. If a patient has a deficiency of a particular vitamin, he needs supplementation. There are several groups of individuals who may have vitamin deficiencies, including people with bowel issues like Celiac disease, Gastric bypass surgery, or pancreatitis. Alcoholics, the elderly, or those on restrictive diets are also at risk of being malnourished. Blood levels for major vitamins can be tested, and any identified deficiency should be corrected. Still, I will repeat my earlier statement: it is always better to get your micronutrients from whole foods or whole food supplements.

WHOLE FOOD SUPPLEMENTS

There is an alternate form of supplement for those who are concerned about vitamins: whole food supplements. A whole food supplement, which is naturally derived from foods, may be in the form of a juice or powder. Being derived from foods, these supplements contain much more nutrition than any vitamin tablet. There are thousands of micronutrients, enzymes, and fiber in foods that are not present in a vitamin tablet. It is this total combination of nutrients that gives the original fruits and vegetables their beneficial properties. After the failures of synthetic vitamins, scientists are now studying the effects of whole food supplements. The results indicate that they may be a good way to supplement one's daily diet when it is not possible to eat multiple servings of fruits or vegetables.

There are many whole food powders or juices on the market, and several research studies demonstrate their benefits. A review of the published studies found that whole food fruit and vegetable concentrates have several heart healthy benefits, including increased blood levels of key nutrients, decreased homocysteine levels, and decreased oxidation in the blood. A separate review confirmed the beneficial effects of fruit and vegetable juices for the prevention of heart disease and some cancers.

Fruit and vegetable juice concentrates increase the total antioxidant capacity in the blood of HIV positive individuals. A concentrate of Japanese apricot was found to suppress infections of the stomach that can later lead to cancer. Japanese-Americans who drank fruit and vegetable juices at least three times a week were 75% less likely to get Alzheimer's disease compared to those who didn't drink juices. Açai berry juice, a potent antioxidant blend, has been found to decrease pain and improve range of motion at 12 weeks. Blood tests also demonstrated mild reductions in inflammation and oxidation markers. Another vegetable powder formulation available as Nanogreens® was found to decrease blood pressure after 90 days.

Encapsulated fruit, vegetable and berry powders under the product name of Juice Plus+® also have been shown to have many health benefits. They promote healthy skin, enhance immune function and antioxidant capacity of the blood, lower homocysteine levels, prevent oxidation of proteins after extreme exercise, reduce symptoms of the common cold, suppress systemic inflammation, help protect DNA, improve the health of gums in persons with periodontal disease, and improve the oxidative status of heavy smokers. Juice Plus+® is the most studied commercial product on the market and has demonstrated multiple health benefits. It is my personal favorite because of the extensive research and health benefits.

In conclusion, there are many healthy diets available and all of the diets presented here have documented health benefits. The hunter-gatherer, DASH, Atkins, Mediterranean, and vegetarian diets can improve your health. Each can be adopted to suit your particular lifestyle and preferences. If it's not possible for you to eat enough fruits and vegetables, I would recommend taking a whole food supplement instead of a traditional vitamin supplement.

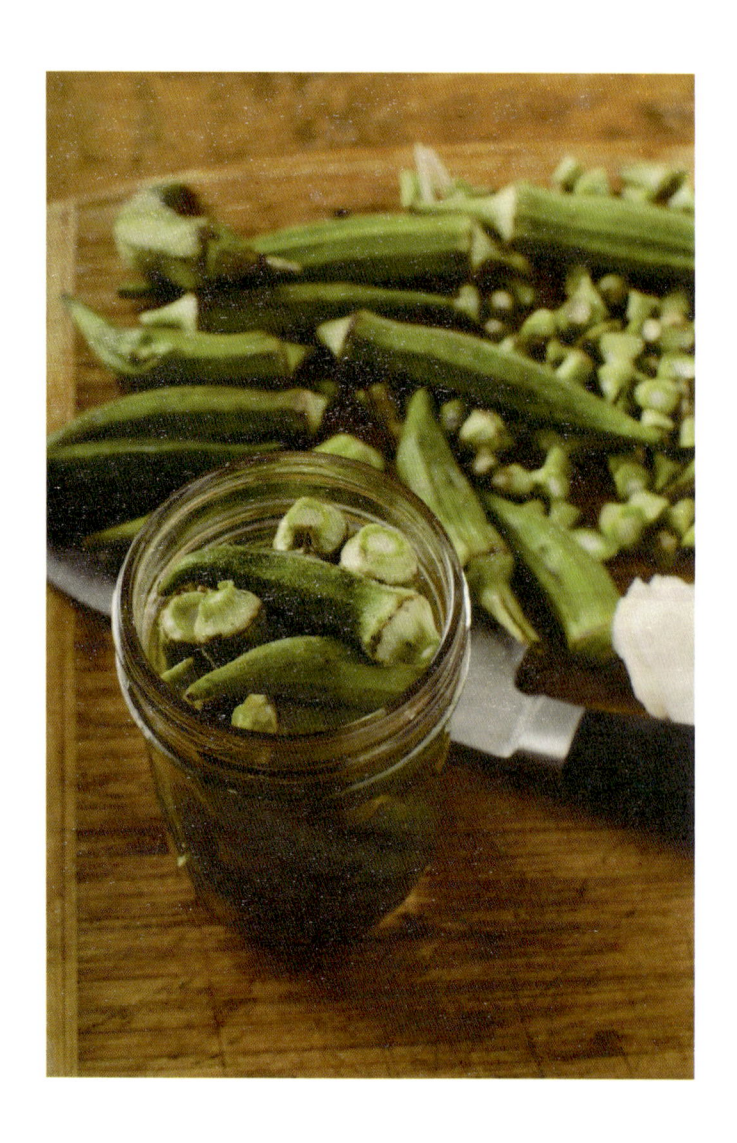

4. PUTTING IT ALL TOGETER

How to develop a healthy diet that fits you

The theme of this book is to demonstrate that healthy eating can lead to reversal or prevention of chronic diseases. This is so important today because medicines are very expensive and do not cure anything. Healthy eating means eating those foods that help all of the body's processes work their best: the genes, DNA repair enzymes, immune system, and stem cells. I am not simply interested in weight loss. It is healthier to remain at a stable weight while eating a healthy diet and exercising than to continuously lose and gain weight. We all have the ability to help our bodies become healthy and it is imperative that we do. It will take some time. There is no quick fix to being healthy; however, if you make changes to your lifestyle based on this book, you will be healthier, feel better, and will probably be able to take less or no medicine.

I briefly outlined the body's processes that keep us healthy: genes, stem cells, and the immune system. We are constantly bombarded by toxins, oxidation, inflammation, and radiation in our environment. Inevitably this brings about damage to our DNA and proteins, but our bodies have fantastic mechanisms to repair damage. All we need to do is give ourselves the necessary tools. Those tools are micronutrients, good fats, good proteins, and good carbohydrates. In the beginning of the book we reviewed current research; now here is the "how to" portion of the book. I'll tell you which fats, proteins, and carbohydrates are good, and where to get all the micronutrients you need. Finally, I'll give you some delicious recipes to follow that will bring these tools into your diet.

FATS

The best fats are monounsaturated, or omega-3 fats. These include olive oil, fish oil, and plant sources, such as flaxseed. There are also omega-3 fats in tree nuts and lean, wild meats. These fats are anti-inflammatory and healthful for your blood vessels and heart, and can even help to prevent cancer. The best olive oil is extra virgin olive oil. It is the most nutritious and delicious. This is the oil that is collected first. Make it a point to get oil described as first press or cold press (although modern methods no longer use a press - instead the oil is separated in a large centrifuge). Lower quality oils will use chemicals to extract the oil, bleach to make it lighter, and deodorizers to remove odors. In the interest of health, avoid eating these chemically treated oils. Olive oil can be added to salads as a dressing, used to sauté vegetables, or sprinkled on pasta. It can be sprinkled on vegetables, fish, or as a dip for bread. This is a much healthier alternative than butter or margarine. My wife's grandmother drank a teaspoon a day, and she stayed healthy and looked great. Here is a new idea I recently discovered: fry your eggs in olive oil! It is delicious and healthy. If you are on a low fat diet, you should limit how much olive oil you use but if you are on a low carbohydrate diet, the amount of olive is not restricted. Sprinkle at will!

FISH OIL

Omega-3 fats are found in highest concentrations in fatty fish like salmon, tuna, sardines, and mackerel. Fish oils can even be taken as a capsule every day. There are many fish capsule brands on the market. The ideal capsule should contain both eicosapentaenoic acid (EPA) and docosahexaenoic acid (DHA) in a 3:2 ratio. The usual daily dose is 1-3 grams daily. Higher doses are sometimes used for certain immune medical conditions, so please consult your doctor if you are thinking about taking higher doses. Many fish species contain mercury, so fish oil capsules are an excellent way to get omega-3 fats without the concern of mercury in the fish.

NUTS AND SEEDS

Flaxseed is another source of omega-3 fats, and it is available whole, ground, or as flaxseed oil. The seed is best since the oil does not contain the beneficial lignans from the coat of the seed. Flaxseed is an excellent source of omega-3 fats and phytoestrogens. For those nutrients and a nice, nutty flavor, put ground flaxseed on cereal, a smoothie, or in muffins.

Tree nuts like pecans, almonds, and walnuts are also a good

source of omega-3 fats, not to mention good carbohydrates and proteins. Tree nuts are a part of the Mediterranean diet and help to make that diet beneficial for heart health. You can add nuts to salads, vegetables, fruit, yogurt, or eat them by the handful. One handful a day is recommended for a Mediterranean-style diet.

PROTEIN

The best sources of proteins, found both in the plant and animal kingdoms, are beans, nuts, fish, poultry, and wild meat. Lean meat is an acceptable substitute, especially if it is grass fed. There are two reasons wild meat is better than domestic beef: first, wild animals are grass fed and their meat contains high levels of omega-3 fats. When cattle are fattened with grains, their meat contains high levels of omega-6 fats, which are inflammatory and lead to chronic diseases. The second reason wild meat is best is that the high activity level of wild animals – that is, the act of running from predators – produces even more of the beneficial omega-3 fats in their meat. True wild meat is difficult to obtain, so you can purchase grass fed, organic beef as an alternate but the healthiest sources of protein are either vegetarian sources of protein, wild meat, wild fish or wild poultry. Grain-fed beef and processed meats like ham, bacon, or cold cuts should be limited to 3 or fewer servings each week.

FISH

Fish is an excellent source of protein that's loaded with omega-3 fats. Wild fish is better than farmed fish, just as it is with beef. You should try to eat at least two meals with fish each week; eating more than that would be even better. All fish contain at least some mercury, a metal that can be absorbed into your body from the foods you eat. High levels affect your nervous system, causing tingling, eye problems, and difficulty with balance and walking, so be mindful of which fish have high levels of mercury. Children and babies in the womb are especially sensitive to mercury, so pregnant women need to be especially cautious about the mercury content of their food. The environmental protection agency and FDA monitor the mercury content of fish. Most people do not have to worry about the health implications of eating fish, but for pregnant women and young children, the FDA has 3 recommendations:

1. Do not eat shark, swordfish, king mackerel, or tilefish. These have the highest mercury content.

2. Eat up to 2 meals each week that include fish with lower mercury content for improved health.

3. Check local advisories about the safety of fish caught in local lakes or rivers.

The FDA publishes tables of levels of mercury in different species of fish to assist you in safe meal planning. The tables are in appendix 1.

POULTRY

Poultry is also a good source of protein, especially if the bird is vegetarian fed. Free range organic chickens are the best. They are a great source to get eggs with a higher omega-3 fat content. There is a lot of discussion about the best way to raise chickens, whether it's caged or free-range. It seems to me that the welfare of the animal is best if it can forage and perform natural activities. In small cages, the animal does not get its full range of exercise. Hormones are not used to raise chickens, but antibiotics have been used since the 1940's, and the safety of this has been questioned. Organic chickens are always preferable if they are available. Chicken must be cooked fully before consumption because the meat can be contaminated with bacteria. Also make sure to wash the cutting board and counter used to prepare poultry before and after use to prevent cross contamination into other foods.

CARBOHYDRATES:

Carbohydrates include simple sugars, starches, and more complex carbohydrates found in grains. Carbohydrates serve as sources of energy for the body, and some carbohydrates are better for the body than others. The glycemic index lists which carbohydrates are better for us, because the glycemic index is a measurement of how high and fast the blood sugar rises after one eats 50 grams of a particular type of carbohydrate. The blood sugar level of the food in question is then measured against a standard, either bread or sugar. Bread and sugar have the highest glycemic indexes because they are absorbed rapidly and cause a quick spike in the blood sugar, therefore their glycemic index is measured as 100 and other foods are measured against them. A slowly absorbed carbohydrate will produce a lower glycemic index. High glycemic index foods cause obesity, metabolic syndrome, and diabetes. Only a very active person or athlete, someone with a high daily caloric usage, should eat a lot of carbohydrates. Sedentary people who eat too many carbohydrates will gain weight. Watch the amount and type of carbohydrate in your diet.

There is a list of foods, and their glycemic indexes and glycemic loads in appendix 2. This is only a partial list and not every food is included. What is the difference between glycemic index and glycemic load? The glycemic load takes into account the serving size of the food. Most foods with a high glycemic index will have a reasonable glycemic load but pay attention to the serving size. The serving sizes are much smaller than those found in the typical American diet. If you eat foods with a high glycemic index, try to stay within the small serving size listed.

Finally, the glycemic index of foods is affected by other foods eaten at the same time. Proteins and fats will slow digestion and decrease the glycemic index of a particular food. It is difficult to determine the glycemic load of an entire meal. As a general rule, I would recommend eating low glycemic index foods as part of a low carbohydrate diet.

Unfortunately, glycemic index and glycemic load listings are not normally available on food packaging. Food manufacturers will only list the amount of carbohydrates per serving. However, this number is important, too. Most people should eat about 200 grams of carbohydrate each day. This number will vary depending on your activity level, age, and whether or not one is following a low carbohydrate diet. The quantity of carbohydrates eaten is as important as glycemic index: too many carbohydrates lead to weight gain. One must count carbohydrates to maintain one's weight.

The basic serving size of a carbohydrate is 15 grams. One slice of bread is 15 grams, rice and potatoes have 30 grams. In the next chapter we will discuss how many carbs one should eat each day. Here is a table with the carbohydrate content of some common foods.

CARBOHYDRATE CONTENT OF COMMON FOODS

Food	Serving	Carbohydrates
Bread	1 slice	15 grams
Bagel	1	40 grams
Cereals	½ cup	15 grams
Donut	1	30 grams

Pasta	1 cup	30 grams
Rice	½ cup	30 grams
Potato	½ cup	30 grams
Starchy vegetable	½ cup	15 grams
Vegetable	½ cup	5 grams
Fruit, apple/orange	1	15 grams
Fruit juice	½ cup	15 grams
Yogurt, plain	¾ cup	10 grams
Milk	1 cup	10 grams
Soda	12 oz. can	40 grams
Beer	12 oz. can	15 grams
Chocolate bar	1.5 oz.	25 grams

MICRONUTRIENTS:

Micronutrients are the vitamins, minerals and enzymes present in fruits and vegetables. They are necessary for the body's functions to work normally. The major vitamins like vitamin A, B, B-12, C, D, E, K calcium, iron, and potassium are familiar to most of us, but have you heard of quercetin, carotene, lutein, zeaxanthin, selenium, polyphenols, flavonoids, or lycopene? They are found in fruits and vegetables, but only a small fraction of the total nutrition of fruits and vegetables exists in a vitamin tablet. This is why vitamin tablets are inadequate. Each micronutrient has a role and so we should try to eat a great variety of fruits and vegetables to get as many of them as possible into our diets (hint: eat twice as many vegetables as fruits). Here are the sources for micronutrients.

Vitamin A:

Vitamin A is important for vision, cell growth, reproduction, and it helps regulate the immune system to fight infections. Vitamin A is made from other nutrients in both animals and plants. In animals, pre-vitamin A is called retinol. In plants, pre-vitamin A is called carotenoid. Beta-carotene is the most active carotenoid. Vitamin A from animal sources includes liver, milk, and fortified foods. Carotenoids from plants include carrots, sweet potatoes, green leafy vegetables (like spinach), kale, mango, apricots, and other darkly colored vegetables. The recommended daily allowance (RDA) is 700-900 international units (IU).

Vitamin B-6:

Vitamin B-6, also known as pyridoxine, is a coenzyme, helping more than 100 enzymes function in the body. It is necessary for the production of neurochemicals in the brain, for regulation of sugar production, for immune system function, and to make red blood cells. Vitamin B-6 is found in fish, beef, liver, and other organ meats, chickpeas, starchy vegetables, potatoes, and non-citrus fruits. The RDA is 1.3-1.5mg daily for adults.

Vitamin B-12:

Vitamin B-12, or cobalamin, is a cofactor that helps enzymes work. It is necessary for red blood cell development, neurologic function and DNA synthesis. B-12 is found in fish, meat, poultry, eggs, milk, and other dairy products. The RDA for vitamin B-12 is 2.4 micrograms daily. Strict vegans who eat no animal products should take a vitamin B-12 supplement to compensate for the lack of B-12 in a plant-only diet.

Vitamin C:

Vitamin C, or ascorbic acid, is found in a variety of foods. Vitamin C is necessary for the production of connective tissues and collagen, L-carnitine, and certain neurotransmitters. It plays an important role in wound healing. Vitamin C is also an important antioxidant. The best sources of vitamin C are citrus fruits, tomatoes, potatoes, red and green peppers, kiwifruits, broccoli, strawberries, Brussels sprouts, and cantaloupe. The RDA for vitamin C is 75-90mg daily.

Vitamin D:

Vitamin D is a fat-soluble vitamin that is necessary for absorption of calcium and bone health. Vitamin D also helps genes perform their function properly, including modulation of cell growth, neuromuscular function, immune system function, and reduction of inflammation. Vitamin D is naturally produced when the skin is exposed to the sun. Other sources include fatty fish, cod liver oil, or supplemented foods. The RDA for vitamin D is 600 IU daily. Many experts believe higher blood levels are important for health and recommend doses as high as 4000-6000 IU daily to get the blood level up to 60-80 nmol/L.

Vitamin E:

Vitamin E exists in eight different forms, but the alpha-tocopherol is the form measured in blood tests. Vitamin E is an antioxidant. It also has a role in immune system function, cell signaling, regulation of gene expression, some other metabolic processes, dilation of blood vessels, and inhibiting platelet functions. Vitamin E is found in nuts, seeds, and vegetable oils, green leafy vegetables, and fortified grains. The RDA for vitamin E is 15mg daily for adults.

Vitamin K:

Vitamin K, also known as phylloquinone, is a very important vitamin for blood clotting, bone health, and for blood vessel health. Warfarin (Coumadin), a common blood thinner, works by blocking the action of vitamin K. If you are taking warfarin, you need to be careful how much vitamin K you eat. Vitamin K is found in green vegetables like collard greens, spinach, broccoli, Brussels sprouts, cabbage, lettuce, asparagus, beans, soybean oil, and canola oil. The RDA for vitamin K is 90-120 micrograms daily.

Folic Acid:

Folic acid, also known as folate or vitamin B-9, is a water-soluble vitamin that is found in many foods. Cells require folic acid in order to reproduce, because it is a necessary ingredient in making DNA and RNA. It also helps in repair of damaged DNA, is needed for production of red blood cells, and helps in the regulation of the amino acid homocysteine. Folate is found in green leafy vegetables, citrus fruits, dried beans, peas, and supplemented grains and flour. The RDA for folate is 600 micrograms daily.

Selenium:

Selenium is a mineral that is necessary for good health, and only a small amount is needed to get the beneficial health effects. It is incorporated into proteins where it acts as an important antioxidant. It also helps with thyroid function and the immune system. Plants are the major source of selenium, but it is also found in fish. The amount of selenium in plants varies depending on the selenium levels of the soil in which the plant was grown. The highest levels are in Brazil nuts, but tuna, cod, turkey, beef, and chicken also contain selenium. The RDA for selenium is 55 micrograms daily.

Zinc:

Zinc is an essential mineral that is present in some foods and may be found in some over-the-counter cold medicines. Zinc is active in several cellular functions through its association with enzymes. It is necessary for immune function, protein synthesis, wound healing, synthesis of DNA, and cell division. It is also necessary for the proper function of the senses of taste and smell. Oysters contain the most zinc, but it can be found in red meat, poultry, beans, nuts, whole grains, dairy products, and fortified cereals. The RDA for zinc is 8-11mg daily.

Thiamin:

Thiamin is an enzyme cofactor that is essential in metabolism of glucose and amino acids to maintain antioxidant status, and for the health of nerves. A deficiency of thiamin causes diseases of the nerves and heart failure. Alcoholics are at risk for deficiency. Thiamin is found in yeast, whole grains and supplemented foods. The RDA for thiamin is 1.1-1.2mg daily.

Riboflavin:

Riboflavin, or vitamin B-2, is necessary for cell growth and metabolism. It is present in small amounts in most plant and animal foods. The best sources include eggs, lean meats, milk, broccoli, and enriched breads and cereals. The RDA for riboflavin is 1.1-1.3mg daily.

Niacin:

Niacin, or vitamin B-3, is necessary for metabolism, production of steroid hormones and repair of DNA. The main sources of niacin are meat, fish, and nuts, but milk and eggs also contain small amounts. The RDA for niacin is 60mg daily.

Pantothenic acid:

Pantothenic acid, or vitamin B-5, is necessary for growth, reproduction and energy production. It helps the body use cholesterol, and maintains the health of the gut. The best dietary sources of pantothenic acid are beef, chicken, eggs, tomato products, broccoli, potatoes, and whole grains. The RDA for pantothenic acid is 5mg daily.

Biotin:

Biotin, known as vitamin H, is a component of enzymes that help break down fats and metabolize proteins. Biotin is found in small amounts in many foods, and is made by bacteria in the gut. Deficiency of biotin is very rare and is characterized by thinning of hair, red scaly rash, depression, tingling in hands and feet, and hallucinations. There is no RDA for biotin.

PHYTOCHEMICALS:

Phytochemicals are compounds produced in plants that have broad biological activities, and are most beneficial due to their epigenetic effects. These compounds have multiple six-sided benzene rings that are called polyphenols, and flavonoids are the most important single group of polyphenols in plants. There are five thousand different types of flavonoids. The different types include flavones, flavonols, flavanones, catechins, proanthocyanidins, anthocyanins, and isoflavones.

Flavones:

The flavones include apigenin and luteolin. They prevent overgrowth of cells and the formation of blood vessels – two processes critical for the formation of cancer. Flavones have been found to inhibit tumor cells. They are found in whole grains, green leafy vegetables, celery, celery hearts, peppers, spinach, green tea and herbs.

Flavonols:

The flavonols include quercetin, kaempferol, myricetin, and isorhamnetin. Quercetin, the most widely studied, is a potent antioxidant and also has beneficial effects on the blood vessels. The sources of flavonols include onions, kale, cocoa, broccoli, blueberries, spinach, blackberries, tea, celery, beans, lettuce, grapefruit, and tomatoes.

Flavanones:

Flavanones are the major flavonoid in citrus fruits and include naringenin, hesperitin, and eriodictyol. They have anti-inflammatory and anti-cancer actions. They are found in oranges, tangerines, mandarins, grapefruit, lemons, and limes. A note of caution: the flavonoids in grapefruit are unique and interact with many medicines, consult your doctor to learn if any of your medications might interact with grapefruit juice.

Catechins:

The catechins are flavan-3-ols and include catechin, epicatechin,

epicatechin-3-gallate, and epigallo-catechin-3-gallate (EGCG). They are found in green tea, black tea, chocolate, blackberries, and apples. EGCG in green tea is one of the most widely studied flavonoids. It is an anti-oxidant, but also has epigenetic effects and helps to turn on anti-cancer genes. Studies are underway to see how well it can prevent cancer. It may also prevent heart disease.

Proanthocyanidins:

Proanthocyanidins, also known as condensed tannins, are one of the most abundant compounds in plants. They are anti-oxidants and help protect cells. They are thought to prevent cancer and chronic diseases. They prevent oxidation of lipids, inhibit platelet function, and inhibit cancer cells. They are found in fruits, berries and chocolate, including blueberries, cranberries, apple, peaches, plums, sorghum, pinto beans, red beans, kidney beans, hazelnuts, pecans, pistachios, and almonds.

Anthocyanins:

Anthocyanins give plants their blue, purple, and red colors. They include cyaniding, delphinidin, peonidin, petunidin, malvidin, and pelargonidin. They assist in the health of blood vessels, and vision.

They have anti-cancer effects and are anti-oxidants. Anthocyanins can be found in elderberry, chokeberry, blueberry, blackberry, cranberry, cherry, raspberry, strawberry, plums, nectarines, peaches, red leaf lettuce, and apples.

Isoflavones:

Isoflavones include genistein and diadzein and are found primarily in legumes like soybeans. The benefits of soybeans are many, including improvement in blood cholesterol, and reducing the risk of heart disease, breast cancer, and prostate cancer, especially if eaten early in life. There are multiple studies showing that isoflavones inhibit the growth of tumor cells. They may also help preserve bone strength.

Isoprenoids (lycopene):

Lycopene is an excellent anti-oxidant. It also helps modulate cell growth and has been found to decrease the risk of cancer, especially prostate cancer, reduce heart disease, and macular degeneration. It can be found in tomatoes, carrots, yams, cantaloupe, spinach, sweet potatoes, watermelon, citrus fruit, pumpkin, apricots, mango, and kale.

Saponins:

Saponins bind bile acids, preventing cholesterol reabsorption, thus reducing cholesterol levels. It has been found to inhibit certain cancer cells and help the immune system. They can be found in legumes and beans.

Tocopherols:

Tocopherols are excellent anti-oxidants and inhibit oxidation of blood cholesterol. They also have anti-cancer activity. They are found in green leafy vegetables, nuts, whole grains, and vegetable oil.

Lignans:

Lignans prevent the formation of free oxygen radicals, lower serum cholesterol, and prevent oxidation of blood lipids. They have been found to reduce the risk of heart disease and breast cancers. They are found in oil seeds like flax, soy, rapeseed, whole grains, legumes, and berries.

Resveratrol:

Resveratrol has many activities: anti-oxidant, antiproliferative, inhibition of cancer cell growth, and metastasis. Resveratrol is heart healthy and prevents cancers. It can be found in grapes and red wine.

ALLYL S-COMPOUNDS:

These amino acid based compounds include diallyl disulfide and allicin. They inhibit human cancer cells, and inhibit cholesterol production. These compounds are found in garlic, onions, leeks, and chives.

Isothiocyanates:

Sulforaphane is an isothyocyanate that has anti-cancer activity. It induces the production of enzymes that breakdown cancer-causing substances (carcinogens). It can also inhibit the activation of carcinogens. Isothyocyanates are found in cruciferous vegetables like broccoli, cauliflower, kale, and Brussels sprouts.

Indoles:

Indole-3-carbinol is a substance that regulates estrogen production and activity. It also inhibits cancers cell growth and has been found to help prevent cancers. Indoles are found in cruciferous vegetables like broccoli, cauliflower, kale, and Brussels sprouts.

Lactoferrin:

Lactoferrin is a protein found in milk. It stimulates beneficial bacteria in the colon and increases the production of growth factors for immune cells. Lactoferrin stimulates the immune system, inhibits bacteria, and aids in healing of gastrointestinal wounds.

Linoleic Acid:

Linoleic acid is a fatty acid found in dairy products and cheeses. It reduces cell growth, improves lipid levels, and increases the breakdown of fats and fatty acids. It is helpful to reduce the risk of cancer, heart disease and obesity.

Linolenic Acid:

Linolenic Acid is a plant-derived fatty acid. It decreases bad cholesterol levels and helps prevent heart disease. It is found in green leafy vegetables, flaxseed, and walnuts.

Omega-3 fatty acids:

Eicosapentaenoic acid (EPA)/Docosahexaenoic acid (DHA) is a fatty acid with multiple health benefits. It improves cholesterol levels, prevents blood clots, and decreases inflammation. It helps prevent heart disease, reduce cholesterol, and lowers inflammation. Omega-3 fatty acids are found in salmon, tuna, other ocean fish, olive oil, and canola oil.

Prebiotics:

Prebiotics support the growth of beneficial bacteria in the colon. These bacteria improve the immune system, protect the body from infections, and modulate lipid metabolism. Prebiotics include garlic, asparagus, chicory, barley, and oatmeal.

Probiotics:

Probiotics are living bacteria that are beneficial for bowel health. They stimulate the immune system, prevent diarrhea, and have anti-cancer effects. The probiotic bacteria include lactobacilli and bifidobacteria, and are found in fermented dairy products, such as yogurt and kefir.

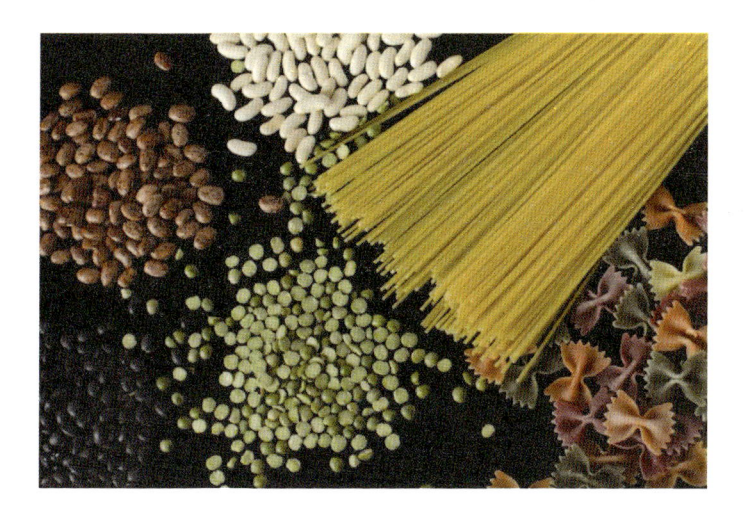

APPENDIX 1: MERCURY CONTENT IN COMMERCIAL FISH

These fish have the highest content of mercury per part. Pregnant women and young children should avoid these fish:

Species	Mercury (parts per million)
Mackerel King	0.73
Shark	0.979
Swordfish	0.995
Tilefish (Gulf of Mexico)	1.45

Source: FDA 1990-2010, "National Marine Fisheries Service Survey of Trace elements in the Fishery Resource" report 1978

"The Occurrence of mercury in the Fishery Resources of the Gulf of Mexico" report 2000

These fish have lower levels of mercury and can be eaten 2 or more times per week:

Species	Mercury (parts per million)
Catfish	0.25
Cod	0.111
Crab	0.065
Crawfish	0.033
Haddock	0.055
Herring	0.084
Lobster (spiny)	0.081
Mackerel, Atlantic	0.093
Mullet	0.050
Oyster	0.012
Perch (ocean)	0.121
Salmon	0.022
Sardine	0.013
Scallop	0.003
Shrimp	0.009

Squid	0.023
Tilapia	0.013
Trout (freshwater)	0.071
Tuna	0.128
Whitefish	0.089

Source: FDA 1990-2010, "National Marine Fisheries Service Survey of Trace elements in the Fishery Resource" report 1978

"The Occurrence of mercury in the Fishery Resources of the Gulf of Mexico" report 2000

Mercury Levels of these Fish are moderate:

Species	Mercury (parts per million)
Bass, saltwater striped	0.152
Bass, Chilean	0.354
Bluefish	0.368
Grouper	0.448
Halibut	0.241
Lobster (Northern)	0.107
Marlin	0.485
Orange Roughy	0.571
Perch	0.150
Snapper	0.166
Tuna, Albacore	0.358
Tuna, Bigeye	0.689
Tuna, Yellow fin	0.354
Weakfish, Sea trout	0.235

Source: FDA 1990-2010, "National Marine Fisheries Service Survey of Trace elements in the Fishery Resource" report 1978

"The Occurrence of mercury in the Fishery Resources of the Gulf of Mexico" report 2000

APPENDIX 2: GLYCEMIC INDEX OF SELECTED FOODS

Bakery Products	Glycemic Index	Glycemic Load/ serving size
Chocolate Cake	38	20/ 4 oz.
Vanilla Cake	42	24/ 4 oz.
Croissant	67	17/ 2 oz.
Muffin	54	14/ 2 oz.
Pancakes	67-100	22-39/ 3 oz.
Waffles	76	10/ 1.2 oz.

Beverages	Glycemic Index	Glycemic Load/ serving size
Cola	63	16/ 8 oz.
Apple juice	40	12/ 8 oz.
Cranberry juice	68	24/ 8 oz.
Orange juice	50	13/ 8 oz.
Tomato juice	38	4/ 8 oz.
Gatorade	78	12/ 8 oz.

Quik	41	4/ 8oz

Breads	Glycemic Index	Glycemic Load/ serving size
Bagel	72	25/ 2.5 oz.
Baguette	95	15/ 1 oz.
Oat-bran	50	9/ 1 oz.
Rye	50	5/ 1 oz.
Wheat, whole	52	10/ 1 oz.
Wheat, white flour	70	10/ 1 oz.
Wonder bread	75	10/ 1 oz.

Breakfast Cereals	Glycemic Index	Glycemic Load/ serving size
All Bran	40	9/ 1 oz.
Cheerios	74	15/ 1 oz.
Coco Puffs	77	20/ 1 oz.
Cornflakes	92	24/ 1 oz.
Cream of Wheat	70	20/ 1 oz.
Fruit Loops	70	18/ 1 oz.
Golden Grams	71	18/ 1 oz.
Grape Nuts	75	16/ 1 oz.
Life	66	15/ 1 oz.
Muesli	50	10/ 1 oz.
Oatmeal	75	17/ 8 oz.
Oatmeal, quick oats	65	17/ 8 oz.

Grains	Glycemic Index	Glycemic Load/ serving
Barley	25	11/ 5 oz.
Buckwheat	54	16/ 5 oz.
Cornmeal	69	9/ 5 oz.
Corn, sweet	53	17/ 5 oz.
Couscous	65	23/ 5 oz.
Rice, white	64	23/ 5 oz.
Rice, long grain	56	23/ 5 oz.
Rice, brown	55	18/ 5 oz.
Wheat	48	14/ 2 oz. dry
Semolina	55	6/ 5 oz.
Wheat, cracked	48	12/ 5 oz.

Dairy Products	Glycemic Index	Glycemic Load/ serving
Custard	43	7/ 3.5 oz.
Ice cream	60	8/ 2 oz.
Milk	27	3/ 8 oz.
Pudding	44	7/ 3.5 oz.
Yogurt, low fat	31	9/ 3.5 oz.
Soy milk	44	8/ 8 oz.

Fruit	Glycemic Index	Glycemic Load/ serving
Apple	38	6/ 1 apple
Apple juice	40	11/ 8 oz.
Apricot, dried	31	9/ 2 oz.
Banana	52	12/ 1 banana
Fruit Cocktail	55	9/ 4 oz.
Grapefruit	25	3/ 1 small

Grapefruit juice	48	9/ 8 oz.
Grapes	46	8/ 4 oz.
Kiwi	53	6/ 4 oz.
Orange	42	5/ 1 orange
Orange juice	52	12/ 8 oz.
Peaches	42	5/ 1 peach
Peaches, canned	38	4/ 4 oz.
Pear	38	4/ 1 pear
Pineapple	59	7/ 4 oz.
Plums	39	5/ 1-2 plums
Watermelon	72	4/ 4 oz.

Legumes and Peas	**Glycemic Index**	**Glycemic Load/ serving**
Baked Beans	48	7 per ½ cup
Beans	29	9 per ½ cup
Black-eyed Peas	42	13 per ½ cup
Butter Beans	31	6 per ½ cup

Chick Peas	28	8 per ½ cup
Navy Beans	38	12 per ½ cup
Kidney Beans	28	7 per ½ cup
Lentils	30	5 per ½ cup
Peas	22	2 per ½ cup
Pinto Beans	39	10 per ½ cup
Soya Beans	18	1 per ½ cup
Split Peas	32	6 per ½ cup

Pasta	Glycemic Index	Glycemic Load/serving
Capellini	45	20 per ¾ cup
Fettuccine	40	18 per ¾ cup
Gnocchi	68	33 per ¾ cup
Linguini	52	23 per ¾ cup
Macaroni	47	23 per ¾ cup
Ravioli	39	15 per ¾ cup
Spaghetti	40	18 per ¾ cup

Tortellini	50	10 per ¾ cup
Vermicelli	35	16 per ¾ cup

Nuts	Glycemic Index	Glycemic Load/ serving
Cashew	22	3 per ¼ cup
Peanuts	14	1 per ¼ cup
Popcorn	72	8 per 1/8 cup

Potato	Glycemic Index	Glycemic Load/ serving
Potato, baked	85	26 per 2/3 cup
Potato, boiled	50	14 per 2/3 cup
Potato, mashed	75	15 per 2/3 cup
Potato, new	57	12 per 2/3 cup
Potato, Sweet	61	17 per 2/3 cup

Adapted from: Kay Foster-Powell, Suzanna HA Holt, Janette C. Brand-Miller. International table of glycemic index and glycemic load values: 2002 Am J Clin Nutr 2002;76:5-56

5. MY THOUGHTS ON WHAT MAKES A HEALTHFUL DIET

How much should you eat?

First, determine how many calories you should eat each day. One general rule is to place a 0 after your ideal weight - that is how many calories you should be eating. If my ideal weight is 200 pounds, then I should eat 2,000 calories a day to maintain that weight. A more accurate way is to look at this table of the estimated daily dietary calories needed to maintain caloric balance.

Age	Sedentary Male	Active Male	Sedentary Female	Active Female
21	2400	3000	2000	2400
31	2400	3000	1800	2200
41	2200	2800	1800	2200
51	2200	2800	1600	2200
61	2000	2600	1600	2000
71	2000	2600	1600	2000

Source: myplate.gov

Once you know how many calories you should be eating, the next step is to break this down into the three macronutrients: protein, carbohydrates, and fat. Each particular diet plan has a ratio of these three components. The numbers are percent of total calories.

Diet	% Fat	% Protein	% Carbohydrate
Standard	30	20-30	40-50
Low Carbohydrate	40-50	20-30	30
Athletes	20	20-30	50-60

It's easy to determine the fat calories allowed in your particular diet plan – simply multiply the calories by the percentage of fat calories in your column. For example, a standard diet would multiply 1,800 calories by the 30% figure found in the table, and 540 is the result. That's the number of calories from fat allowed for that diet.

Protein and carbohydrates need to be converted to grams. For protein, take your weight in pounds and divide by 3.7 to learn how many grams of protein you should eat each day. The CDC recommends women over the age of 19 eat 46 grams of protein each day and men eat 56 grams of protein. The RDA for protein is 0.35 grams per pound of weight. So if you weigh 140 pounds, multiply by 0.35 to get the answer. You should eat 49 grams of protein.

For carbohydrates, multiply the total daily calories by the percentage of carbohydrates associated with your diet. For an 1,800 calorie diet, multiply by 0.5 for standard diets, 0.3 for low carbohydrate and 0.6 for athletes. To convert calories of carbohydrates to grams of carbohydrates, divide by 4. This gives you grams of carbohydrates to eat each day. This table presents this information for an 1,800 calorie diet. The numbers will vary according to the total calories allowed.

Type of diet	Fat calories	Protein	Carbohydrate
1800 standard	540 calories	0.35 X wt.	180-225 grams
1800 Low Carb	720-900 calories	0.35 X wt.	135 grams
1800 Athlete	360 calories	0.5 X wt.	225-270 grams

What is a healthful diet, exactly?

I've presented information about many things in this book. We discussed epigenetics and how it relates to disease. We discussed healthy foods that help cells function properly, the immune system, stem cells, and some of the healthiest diets with scientific studies demonstrating their benefits. Now the question is, what diet should you follow? What fits your personality better: Paleothic, low carbohydrate, DASH, Mediterranean, vegetarian, or a combination? They are all healthful and all have scientific studies backing them up. Low carbohydrate diets are an excellent way to lose weight quickly. It's possible to adjust any of these diets to include lower carbohydrates. My personal opinion is that low carbohydrates are essential to a healthful diet. We have a lot of diseases because of processed sugar and carbohydrates. Whole-grains are healthier, but still should be limited. The Paleo and Atkins diets are low carbohydrate by design, but you can also lower the carbohydrate content of a vegetarian or Mediterranean diet. Whichever diet you choose, there are important key points that you should follow regarding protein, carbohydrates, fats, and micronutrients.

Protein:

The original Atkins concept was flawed. It did not discriminate between types of fat or meat. This diet may not be safe if it involves large amounts of saturated fats and red meat. Saturated fats, red meat, and processed meats like bacon and ham cause inflammation and lead to an increased risk of cancer. The hunter-gatherer diet includes a higher proportion of meat than the other diets, but does not cause heart disease because it specifies that the meat be lean and preferably wild. The amount of meat eaten can increase if the meat is lean, wild meat. With this fact in mind, the Atkins diet has been amended to include healthier forms of proteins and fats. Fish and chicken are also excellent forms of animal protein. Wild fish is best and has been found to be quite beneficial (as long as you avoid high mercury content). Chicken and turkey are also lean forms of animal protein. They are healthful, too, as long as they are not battered and fried. Plant forms of protein are especially healthy and are a great alternative for eating meat. Any diet can be supplemented with vegetarian meals and I highly recommend this option, which also helps stretch a food budget as meat and fish prices rise each year.

Carbohydrates:

Carbohydrates are important for energy, especially if you are very active. The reason we have an obesity problem in this country is most people lead sedentary lives and don't need many carbohydrates. We eat too many carbohydrates, including 180 pounds of sugar each year in our food and drinks. Whether you are on a low carbohydrate or normal carbohydrate diet, you need to watch the glycemic index to avoid high sugar intake. To lose weight, decrease carbohydrate intake. If you are eating to maintain a weight level, choose low glycemic index foods to maintain your health. High glycemic index foods will tend to cause the problems we discussed: obesity, metabolic syndrome, diabetes, and heart disease. If you like to eat sweet foods, it may not be easy to give up sugar at first, but it is vitally important for your long-term health. Take your time and decrease the sugars slowly if you need to. Try low glycemic sweeteners as an alternative to sugar. For example, agave syrup has one of the lowest glycemic indexes of any sweetener. Here is a list of common sweeteners and their glycemic index:

Type of Sweetener	Average Glycemic Index
Glucose	100
Fructose (Fruit)	19
Sucrose (table sugar)	68
Honey	55
Maple syrup	68
Lactose	46
Agave syrup	10-11
Sugar free sweeteners	0

Diabetics must count carbohydrates to keep their disease in control. This is a necessity for anyone with diabetes, but there is no reason you have to wait until you are diagnosed with diabetes to watch your carbohydrates. Remember, diabetes is preceded by metabolic syndrome and metabolic syndrome is caused by consuming too many high-glycemic foods. Anyone who is overweight, has high triglycerides, high cholesterol, or high blood pressure is on their way to becoming diabetic. They should be on a low carbohydrate diabetes type diet to prevent diabetes. Diabetes runs in families, so if you have family members with adult onset diabetes, you need to reduce your glycemic load before you get diabetes. Diseases are always easier to prevent than to treat after they occur.

A typical serving of a carbohydrate is 15 grams. The number of servings allowed varies in each diet. To keep the glycemic index low, substitute whole grain breads for white bread, or wheat bread and brown rice for white rice. Pasta has a lower glycemic index than bread because it is so dense. Serve it al dente (chewy not mushy) to keep the glycemic index low. Sugary soft drinks, cake, pie, cookies, and other dessert should be a rare treat, not a regular food item. Remember, Americans used to eat only one pound of sugar each year.

Micronutrients:

Every healthy diet has one thing in common: fruits and vegetables. They are loaded with vitamins, minerals, and phytonutrients. Although the government only recommends five servings a day of fruits and vegetables, healthy diets like the DASH, Mediterranean, vegetarian, and Paleolithic include many more servings. That is why they prevent and reverse diabetes and heart disease. Remember to mix it up and get a sample from all the colors and types of vegetables and fruits each week. If you can't manage to include enough fruits and vegetables, add a whole food supplement. There are some really impressive whole food supplements on the market with research to back their claims. Juice Plus+® has the most research of any supplement and is my personal choice. If all else fails, grab a V8® (the low sodium kind, of course).

Here is a review of the diets I presented.

A Paleolithic Diet is based on lean meat, fish, fruits, leafy and cruciferous vegetables, root vegetables, eggs, and nuts. No dairy products, grains, flour, salt or sugar. Technically, no oils, butter, or margarine should be used, but most recipes I see use these. After all, the meal has to be edible. If followed closely, the resulting diet is high protein, low carbohydrate, low fat, and it is high in vegetables and fruit. There was no tea, coffee or alcohol in the Paleolithic era. It's up to you if you want to add tea or coffee. The meals are 50-60% meat and the rest is vegetables, fruits, eggs, and nuts. There is no counting of calories or carbohydrates necessary.

The Mediterranean diet is based on whole grain cereals, low-fat dairy products, potatoes, legumes, vegetables, fruits, fatty fish, olive oil, and canola oil. Red meat is limited, poultry is okay. Here are typical menu items each week. Legumes: eat daily, Fruit: 2.5 cups daily, vegetables: 2 cups daily, fish: more than twice a week, nuts: a handful each day, meat and poultry: less than 4 ounces daily, dairy: 2 cups of low fat daily, wine: optional (one glass for women or two glasses for men), fats: primarily olive oil, eggs: fewer than four each week. You will need to watch calories and carbohydrates if you are watching your weight. The lesson we learned from Greece is a high fat diet is not detrimental to your health as long as they are omega-3 fats.

The DASH diet is based on low salt, increased fruits and vegetables, low fat, and small amounts of lean meat. This is what a DASH diet would look like based on 2,000 calories a day: whole grains, 7-8 each day; fruits, 4-5 each day; vegetables, 4-5 each day; low fat or nonfat dairy foods, 2-3 each day; lean meats, fish, poultry, two or less; nuts, seeds, legumes, 4-5 per week; fats and sweets, limited.

There are a wide variety of vegetarian and vegan diets. You can simply leave out the red meat and poultry, some even exclude fish. If you eat dairy and eggs as well, you are following a lacto-ovo vegetarian diet. If you refrain from all animal foods, meats, dairy and eggs, you are following a vegan diet. There are no hard rules about what to eat besides these, but you would need to count calories and carbohydrates, otherwise you could gain weight on a vegetarian diet. I would make sure to follow the same rules about glycemic index, healthy fats, and low sodium. This would be a basic daily menu for each of these diets.

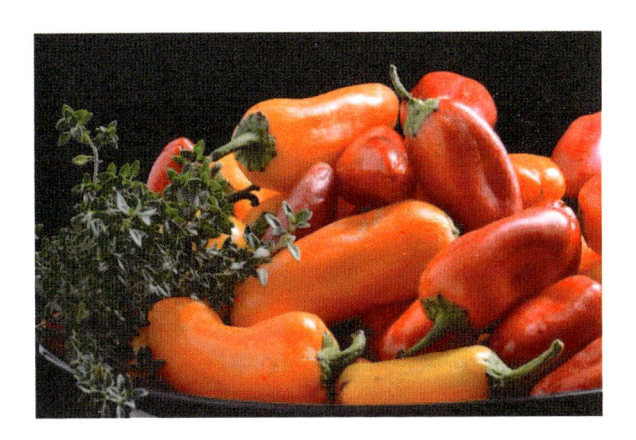

Typical Meals Based on Diet

Paleolithic (Hunter-Gatherer)

Breakfast	Lunch	Dinner
2 eggs any style Chicken or turkey 1 cup of fruit Fruit juice, water	Lean meat of choice Green Salad Vegetable of choice	Lean meat of choice Salad Vegetable Fruit

Low Carbohydrate

Breakfast	Lunch	Dinner
2 eggs any style Lean meat 1 cup of fruit Coffee or tea#	Grilled Turkey No bun or just one slice Cheese Pickle	Lean meat Green Salad Vegetable Tea, coffee, water

DASH

Breakfast	Lunch	Dinner
Whole grain cereal Yogurt Whole grain toast 1 cup fruit Juice, coffee or tea#	Vegetable soup Multigrain turkey sandwich Salad or veggie Apple	Lean meat Brown rice Vegetable Salad Grapes

Mediterranean

Breakfast	Lunch	Dinner
Whole grain cereal **Yogurt** **Whole grain toast** **1 cup fruit** **Juice, coffee or tea#**	Grilled fish/lamb Salad/olive oil Dates/figs Whole grain bread	Fish @ Small serving pasta Vegetable Salad, olive oil Fruit Glass red wine

Vegetarian

Breakfast	Lunch	Dinner
Whole grain cereal, **soy milk** **Toast** **Fruit** **Coffee/tea**	Grilled tomato sandwich Salad	Vegetarian chili Bread Salad Fruit

cream ok, low calorie sweetener if needed, @baked, grilled, but not fried

As you can see, the diets are similar in many ways, but different enough that you can pick one that fits your taste. The vegetarian diet could resemble the low carbohydrate, DASH, or Mediterranean diets with the simple exclusion of the meat components. One item that varies in the diets is the amount of carbohydrates. These are the key to either losing or maintaining your weight. Here is a table of some basic carbohydrate counts. This is not a complete list, so you would also want to check the labels on the foods you eat. Remember, look at glycemic index!

CARBOHYDRATE CONTENT OF COMMON FOODS

Dairy	Carbohydrates (grams)
Cheese	0
Milk	15 per glass
Yogurt	15 per serving

Meat/ Fish	Carbohydrates (grams)
Chicken, roasted *	0
Red meat	0

Turkey, roasted*	0
Pork	0
Ham	0
Fish, roasted*	0

*breading adds 15-30 grams carbohydrates

Vegetables	Carbohydrates (grams)/ serving
Beans, boiled	10 per 1 cup
Broccoli	5 per 1 cup
Peas/carrots	10 per 1 cup
Celery	0 per stalk
Cucumber	2 per 1 cup
Okra	5 per 1 cup
Peppers	2 per 1 cup
Potato, baked	30
Soybeans	20 per 1 cup
Spinach	5 per 1 cup

Squash, raw	5 per 1 cup
Squash, cooked	15-20 per 1 cup
Tomato sauce	20 per 1 cup
Tomato, raw	5
Tomato, cooked	10

Soup	Carbohydrates (grams)/ serving
Noodle soup	30-50
Vegetable soup	15 grams

Seeds	Carbohydrates (grams)/ serving
Flaxseed	5 per 1 Tbsp.
Sunflower	5 per 1 oz.
Sunflower	30 per 1 cup

Nuts, not honey roasted	Carbohydrates (grams)/ serving
Almonds	15 per 1 cup
Pecans	15 per 1 cup
Mixed nuts	30 per 1 cup

Grains	Carbohydrates (grams/ 1 cup)
Buckwheat flour	100
Barley flour	100
Couscous	30
Hominy	25
Noodles	40
Oats	100
Rice, wild	35
Rice, white	50
Rice, brown	50
Spaghetti	40

Wheat flour	100
Wheat bran	40

Cereals and Breads	Carbohydrates (grams) / serving
Unsweetened breakfast cereal	25-50 grams
Granola, homemade	15
Granola	65
Bread, white	15 each
Bagel, small	30 each
Bagel, large	70 each
Biscuit	15-30 each
English muffin	30 each
Muffin	30 each
Pancakes	15-30 each
Taco shell	15 each
Tortilla, small	15-30 each

Tortilla, large	40-60 each
Toaster pastry	30 each
Waffles	15-30 each

Dressings, without sugar	Carbohydrates (grams)
Oil/Vinegar	0
Mayonnaise	0

Fruit	Carbohydrates (grams)
Juices	30 per cup
Apple	15
Berries	20 per cup
Orange	15
Grapes	30-50 per cup
Raisins	30 per 1.5 oz.
Watermelon	15 per cup

Tables adapted from Carbohydrate-counter.org

RECIPES:

Here are some basic ideas and recipes to make healthful, great tasting meals. The awesome thing about food is the huge variety of menus possible in any given diet. The combinations of colors, flavors, and textures are endless. Start with some basic ideas and cooking techniques, then feel free to experiment and add flavors to suit your tastes. This is only meant as a guide.

BREAKFAST:

Breakfast is the most important meal of the day. It breaks the fast you had from the night before, it increases your metabolism and that assists in weight loss, but more importantly, it gives you a great start for the day ahead of you. Students, kids, adults, busy executives, and busy mothers all perform better if they get a good start to the day. There are some foods to avoid, though. You don't want a breakfast high in sugar. One of the worst combinations would be a donut or bagel and a glass of juice. This has high carbs and high glycemic index. Talk about a sugar high! Your sugar will skyrocket by 9 AM and crash at 10:30, setting up for a midmorning snack of a sugary muffin at the office, which would lead to another crash before lunchtime....what you eat affects you all day. Sugar highs and lows increase your insulin, insulin resistance, inflammation, and oxidation. The ideal breakfast has some healthy carbs, micronutrients, and protein, with low sodium and low sugar. Here are some great ideas for breakfast.

Smoothie:

Breakfast smoothies are a great way to start the day. They are easy to prepare, fast, and healthful if you make them the correct way. Watch out for smoothies at fast food restaurants. They are loaded with sugar – sometimes more sugar than in a soft drink. The best plan is to make it at home and add the ingredients you like. The possibilities are endless. There are several basic ingredients to a smoothie.

1. Fruit: Most people will start with some sort of fruit for their smoothie. This can be any fruit: apple, orange, peach, pear, plums, strawberries, kiwi, banana, watermelon, cantaloupe, honeydew, berries or any other fruit you can think of. The fruit adds fiber, micronutrients, and sweetness. Once you have adjusted to a no-added sugar lifestyle, you will find the fruit adds just enough sweetness to the smoothie without being too sweet. Using frozen fruit will eliminate the need for ice cubes in many recipes.

2. Liquid: It will be necessary to add some sort of liquid so you can drink your smoothie instead of spoon it out of a cup. There are many possibilities like water, low-fat milk, soy milk, coconut milk, almond milk, or yogurt. You could also use fruit juice, but juice adds lots of carbohydrates. It is better to eat the whole fruit and get its fiber and nutrients.

3. Protein: There is protein in dairy products or soy milk if you choose to use those. Some people also like to add extra protein to their smoothies in the form of whey protein or soy protein, the two most common forms. You can also add amino acids like glutamine, which is a source of protein and is beneficial to your immune system. When you add nuts, you add protein plus a lot of other healthy nutrients, carbohydrates and fats.

4. Nuts: Tree nuts are an excellent source of good carbohydrates, protein, and mono-unsaturated fats. They are great for your heart's health and add a nice "nutty" taste to your smoothie. Try pecans, walnuts, almonds, or other nuts.

5. Vegetables: It may sound unusual in a breakfast shake, but adding vegetables can improve the flavor and adds more nutrition. Some good vegetables include carrots, spinach, lettuce, peas, green beans, broccoli, cauliflower, or peppers. You can vary it based on what flavors you like. Carrots and peas add sweetness, while spinach does not add much flavor. Lettuces can add bitterness, depending on the type of lettuce. Peppers add sweetness or spice depending on the type of pepper.

6. Spirulina: Blue-green algae is an excellent nutrition source and, as you recall, is an excellent food for your stem cells. It will turn any smoothie blue-green, so be prepared for the color!

7. More flavors: Don't forget the spices! They add wonderful flavors and health benefits. Many are antioxidants and have heart protective and anti-cancer benefits. Cinnamon helps to prevent diabetes and improve insulin sensitivity. Clove is a powerful antioxidant. Cacao is a powerful

antioxidant and its polyphenols are heart healthy. It also gives your smoothie a delicious chocolate taste. Cayenne pepper adds a little spice and also has anti-cancer effects. Cumin, a popular spice in the Orient, adds sweetness and a unique flavor. It also has anti-cancer effects. Ginger adds a spicy taste and has been found to have anti-cancer effects. More adventurous people might try a little oregano, rosemary, thyme, or basil. They are excellent anti-oxidants and add unique flavors.

8. Sweetness: Some people prefer sweet smoothies. You have to be mindful of the carbohydrates and the glycemic index, so add only small amounts of sweeteners. I would recommend natural, unprocessed forms of sugars such as whole cane sugar, honey, or agave juice. Agave juice has the lowest glycemic index of these three. Fruit ingredients also sweeten a smoothie, so a fruit smoothie shouldn't require much additional sugar.

9. Other powder: You can also add wheat germ, bee pollen, or flaxseed for other healthy additions to your morning drink.

10. Finally, add ice cubes if needed, then blend. You now have a nutritious, energy-packed drink that will get you to lunch without a midmorning crash. Depending what you add to the smoothie, you will have approximately 50-100 grams of carbohydrates.

Cereals:

Avoid processed cereals, which use grains that have had their bran and germ mechanically removed. The bran and the germ are the parts of the grain that contain nutrients like riboflavin, niacin, thiamin, and iron. In fact, processing removes so much nutrition that cereals need to be fortified with synthetic vitamins. They are then proclaimed nutritious, but the original, whole food is much more healthful. Look for whole grain cereals like granola – but watch the carbohydrate count! Granola is healthful, but also fairly high in carbohydrates. A breakfast with whole grain granola cereal, skim milk, fruit, and yogurt is delicious and contains only 75 carbs.

Fresh fruit of all kinds can be enjoyed any time during the day, but it's especially good during breakfast. Fruit juices have more concentrated sugars and no fiber, so limit the serving to a small glass. Dehydrated fruit has concentrated sugars and more carbohydrates. Tomato juice is also good at breakfast, but be sure it's a low sodium version. An apple, orange, or other fruit has only 15-20 carbs.

Breakfast omelets are delicious and make an excellent meal in a low carbohydrate diet. I love to have omelets because you can include so many other foods in them. You can sauté mushrooms, fresh salsa, herbs, cheese, or a meat. You can add foods and spices to give your omelet the flavor of Tex-Mex, Italian, or Mediterranean. An omelet with sautéed mushrooms, onions, peppers, tomatoes, and cheese is delicious and has fewer than 5 carbs.

If you don't like omelets, you can still enjoy eggs. I used to fry eggs in bacon grease in the traditional Southern way, until I saw a cooking show from Spain on television. They fried their eggs in olive oil. It is a great, healthy idea, and the eggs taste great, too (very low carbs, < 5 grams). Add herbs or fresh basil to give your eggs a wonderful taste.

Pancakes are a tradition in American breakfasts, but read the labels carefully because pancake mixes often incorporate trans-fats to extend shelf life. Select a mix carefully or make your own mix from scratch. Light oils like canola, grape seed, or flaxseed oils can be used, or you can add the whole flaxseed. Flaxseed is very oily and can substitute as a source of oil for baking. Top the pancakes with warmed berries instead of using syrup. (Caution, high carbs! 15-30 grams each pancake).

Muffins are delicious and they are even better if made with whole grain flour. Add flaxseed or wheat germ and enjoy. Old fashioned biscuits and grits have very high carbs and should only be eaten occasionally, or not at all. The carbohydrate count for a muffin is approximately 30 grams.

Fried tomatoes are delicious and can be enjoyed anytime. Put a small amount of olive oil in a pan and add tomatoes, Italian herbs and top with parmigiano reggiano cheese. (Carbs: 10 grams) Add slices of bread to make a fried tomato sandwich. (Carbs: 40-50)

Low fat yogurt with live cultures is delicious and helps your gut and immune system. Add frozen berries or fruit of your choice or granola for a delicious breakfast. (Carbs 50-100 grams)

Blended orange juice tastes better than plain orange juice and adds nutrition. I add frozen raspberries, a teaspoon of cinnamon and 1 teaspoon of cocoa. Put it in a blender and blend with a few ice cubes and voila – it's a delicious fruit smoothie. Fruit juices contain a lot of sugar, so be careful of the amount you are drinking (Carbs: 30-50 grams).

Oatmeal is an excellent way to start the day. Oats are processed just like other grains, so I buy steel cut oatmeal. This preserves the bran, germ and vitamins. I add pecans and honey. It is a whole grain treat (Carbs 65-90).

LUNCH:

In some cultures, lunch is the largest meal of the day and it's followed by a nap. Since most American schedules do not allow for a siesta, we need a light lunch with low carbohydrates. I eat salads or vegetables, and only occasionally add meat. My typical lunch is a salad with olive oil, baked fish, and unsweetened tea. (Very low carbs: < 5 grams) Here are some other great ideas for lunch.

A tomato sandwich is one of my favorites, especially if you use home grown or farm stand tomatoes. I add olive oil, herbs, and cheese and then grill. (Carbs: tomato 5 grams, each slice of bread 15 grams)

Sardines on bread are a great source of omega-3 fats, calcium and vitamin D. You don't have to worry about mercury, because sardines have one of the lowest mercury content levels of any fish. This is one of the best heart healthy fish. (Carbs: 15 grams for the bread)

Soups of all kinds are an excellent source of nutrition. Vegetable soups of all kinds will provide micronutrients. Soups are an excellent vegetarian meal or one can easily add meat, chicken, or sea food. Herbs add flavor and nutrition. Check the labels of store-bought soups for the sodium content. Many soups are high in salt, and the "low salt" varieties may not really have much less sodium. Soups pair well with salads, sandwiches, or just a slice of whole grain or seven-grain bread. (Carbs: 30-50 grams)

A small bowl of pasta with sauce is made better by adding vegetables to the sauce to make pasta primavera. Remember to use olive oil to get the healthy omega-3 fats. Just about anything can be sautéed and added to pasta. There are a variety of sauces like red sauce, white sauce, and pesto and you can add lean meat, poultry or fish. If you are a vegetarian you can add lots of delicious vegetables. (Carbs: 50-100 grams depending on the vegetable and the sauce).

Left-over chicken or turkey can be warmed up and served with all-fruit preserves or cranberries on a bed of lettuce for a low carb treat. (Carbs 15-30 grams)

Organic peanut butter or nut butter can be served with a variety of foods. Serve with apples, pears, celery, or other fruit for a hunter-gatherer lunch. Serve on whole grain toast, and you can add honey to any of these options for some sweetness. (Carbs: 15 grams or 30-40 grams with toast and honey)

A vegetable platter can be served any time. It can be your lunch, a snack, or an appetizer for dinner. A platter of carrots, celery, tomatoes, and edamame (soy beans) is delicious and low in carbohydrates. (Carbs: 15 grams) Avoid the ranch dressing that comes with the platter.

Try a tuna sandwich served opened face with relish, topped with cheese and heated in the oven (Carbs: 15 grams)

DINNER:

Dinner is the largest meal for most people. It is also a very important meal. It is the time when families should sit together and enjoy a meal. As reported in TIME magazine in 2006, sitting together as a family at the dinner table is deeply important for many reasons. Studies show that children who eat with their families are less likely to smoke, use drugs, drink, engage in premarital sex, get depressed, or develop eating disorders. They also score better in school, eat more vegetables, and learn table manners. The most extensive study of family meals to date was published by the National Center on Addiction and Substance Abuse at Columbia University. The CASA study, as it was called, demonstrated that the experience of dining with the family became better the more times a week it was attempted. Those who ate together three or fewer times a week were more likely to watch television instead of talking during dinner. Dinnertime is essential for the development of the family. It is a place for stories, laughter, and the occasional argument, but in the end it forms a tight bond that lasts forever. Don't forget to enjoy food together as a family.

Dinner is typically set up like you see at a restaurant: a main course, sides, dessert and drink. Here are some healthy ideas for each of these courses.

Main course:

Fish is a great source of protein, as it is beneficial for the heart and brain. It can be baked, pan fried in light oil, grilled, smoked, or served over pasta. I like to grill my fish and add herbs and olive oil. It tastes great and is a low carbohydrate item as long as it's not breaded. (Carbs: 0 grams)

Chicken or other poultry is also very healthy. It can be baked, fried, or grilled. It is also a low carbohydrate item as long as there is no breading or stuffing.

Lean meat is a controversial subject. Many studies equate red meat with heart disease and cancer. The data from the hunter-gatherer diet would suggest otherwise as long as the carbohydrates are kept low. There is an increase in cancer risk with processed meats. That includes ham, bacon, or any other salted/smoked meat. Wild meat or grass fed meat is the healthiest. (Carbs: 0 grams)

Vegetarian main courses can include soy, tofu, or beans for the source of protein. There are many ways to cook all of these foods so they seem just like meat. It's easy to have meatless meals. The American standard of a meat and two sides for a meal has become the custom, but it can easily be broken. Some vegetarian main courses may include chili, stews, pasta dishes, sandwiches or a Panini.

Sides:

Pasta side is an excellent side dish because the toppings for the pasta are endless. It can be made as a simple dish with olive oil, tomato sauce or pesto, or it can include vegetables, stews, or meat dishes. (Carbs: 60 grams for one cup of pasta)

Salads are a fantastic way to get your green leafy vegetables and also other vegetables or fruits. Don't stop with iceberg lettuce and a tomato. A wide variety of greens and vegetables can make salad as interesting as you like. This is your chance to stock up on micronutrients. Use an olive oil based dressing with no sugar in it, and the salad becomes a low-carb nutrition powerhouse. (Carbs: 0 grams)

Vegetables can be served in a variety of ways that make them tasty and healthy. They can be baked, sautéed, steamed, or put in soups or stews. Remember to eat 6 or more servings of vegetables every day. (Carbs: 15-30 grams)

DESSERTS:

Desserts are the sweet treat at the end of the meal. It is a little reward for your hard work at trying to keep a healthy lifestyle. A small indulgence does not have to be bad, though. There are many ways to enjoy healthful desserts. This is a great place to add fruit. Dark chocolate is also an excellent addition. The polyphenols in dark chocolate are good for the heart. Yogurt is an excellent, low-sugar alternative to ice cream.

Yogurt with fruit (Carbs 30-50 grams)

Fruit, plain (Carbs: 15 grams)

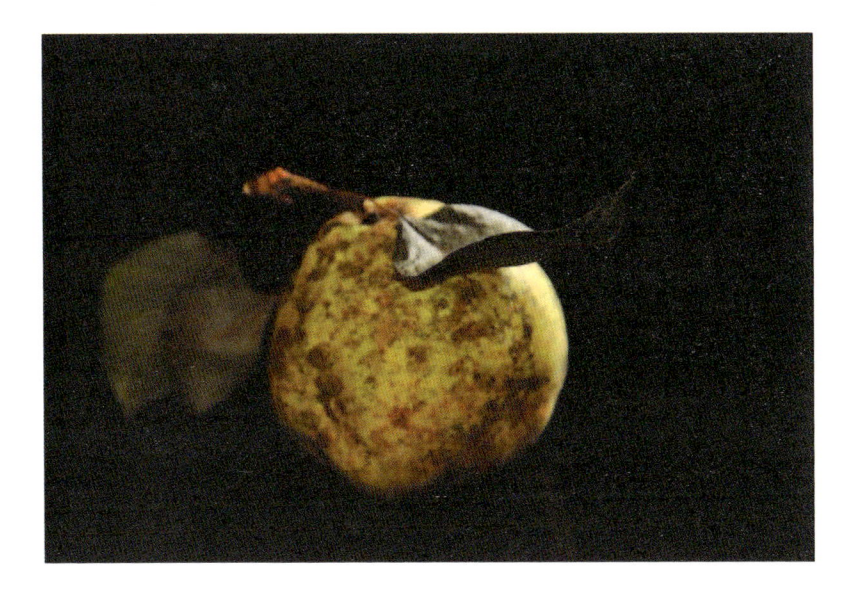

CONCLUSION:

Medicine Free! It's not just a title, it's a way of life. To be truly medicine free, you need to be healthy. To be healthy, all your body's organs and processes must be working correctly. The way to ensure your body works correctly is by healthful living. You have an amazing body that can avoid disease, fight infections and repair itself on a daily basis; all it needs is good nutrition. The best part of a healthful lifestyle is you will cut your dependence on medicines. Medicines are a trap. They treat a symptom but do not cure any chronic diseases. I've demonstrated in this book how certain healthy foods and diets can prevent or reverse disease and break your dependence on medicine. That not only saves you money, it can quite possibly save your life. So now when someone asks "Are you healthy?" You can answer, "Yes, I feel healthy and I am healthy." Let's get going, get some good foods, and start your new healthful lifestyle!

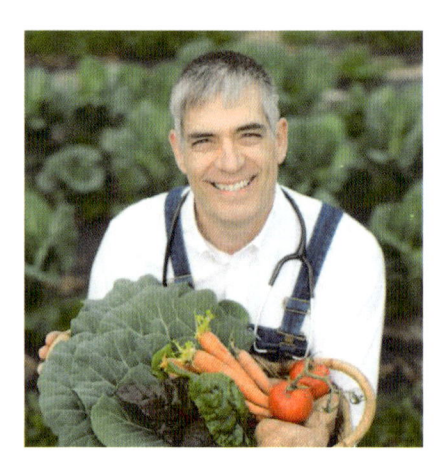

REFERENCES

References Chapter 1:

1. Pray, LA. Discovery of DNA structure and function: Watson and Crick
http://www.nature.com/scitable/topicpage/discovery-of-dna-structure-and-function-watson-397

2. Human Genome Project, nature.com.
http://www.nature.com/scitable/definition/human-genome-project-hgp-112

3. Bose, S. et al. The presence of typical and atypical bcr-abl fusion genes in leukocytes of normal individuals: biologic significance and implications for the assessment of minimal residual disease. Blood 1998;92:3362-3367

4. Stephen Chen, Length of Human DNA Molecule.
http://hypertextbook.com/facts/1998/StevenChen.shtml

5. Rodenhiser, D, Mann, M. et. al. Epigenetics and human disease: translating basic biology into

clinical applications. CMAJ 2006;174(3):341-348

6. Allegrucci C. et al. Epigenetics and the germline. Reproduction 2005;129:137-149

7. Behavior Risk Factor Surveillance System, National Health and Nutrition Survey. www.cdc.gov/nchs/nhanes.htm

8. Obesity, a call to action. The Office of the Surgeon General.
http://www.surgeongeneral.gov/topics/obesity/calltoaction/fact_consequences.htm

9. National Center for Health Statistics.
http://www.cdc.gov/nchs/data/series/sr_10/sr10_249.pdf

10. Cost of Obesity Approaching $300 Billion a year. USA today 1-12-2011

11. Metabolic Syndrome.
http://www.mayoclinic.com/health/metabolic%20syndrome/DS00522

12. Neel, JV. Diabetes mellitus: A "thrifty" genotype rendered detrimental by "progress"? Am J Hum Gen 1962;14(4):353-362

13. Folic Acid Fortification, Centers for Disease Control and Prevention.
http://www.cdc.gov/Features/FolicAcidFortification

14. Ionesco, Ittu, R. et al. Prevalence of severe congenital heart disease after folic acid fortification of grain products: time trend analysis in Quebec, Canada. Medscape.com
http://www.medscape.com/viewarticle/703199

15. Greenberg JA et al. Folic acid supplementation and pregnancy: more than just neural tube defect prevention. Rev Obst Gynecol 2011;4(2):52-59

16. Boucher, O. et al. Neurophysiologic and neurobehavioral evidence of beneficial effects of prenatal omega-3 fatty acid intake on memory function at school age. Am J Clin Nutr 2011;93(5):1025-1037

17. Gilman, MW. Et al. Maternal calcium intake and offspring blood pressure. Circulation 2004;110:1990-1995

18. Toschke, AM. Et al. Early uterine exposure to tobacco-inhaled products and obesity. Am J Epidemiol 2003;158:1068-1074

19. Kaati, G. et al. Cardiovascular and diabetes mortality determined by nutrition during parents' and grandparents' slow growth period. European J Hum Genetics 2002;10:682-688

20. Bertram, C. et al. The maternal diet during pregnancy programs altered expression of the glucocorticoid receptor and type 2, 11β-hydroxysteroid dehydrogenase: potential molecular mechanisms underlying the programming of hypertension in utero. Endo 2001;142(7):2841-2853

21. Lillycrop, L. et al. Dietary protein restriction of pregnant rats induces and folic acid supplementation prevents epigenetic modification of hepatic gene expression in offspring. J Nutr 2005;135:1382-1386

22. Phuc Le, P. et al. Glucocorticoid receptor-dependent gene regulatory networks. PLoS Genetics 2005;1(2):e16

23. Lillycrop, L. et al. Induction of altered epigenetic regulation of the hepatic glucocorticoid receptor in the offspring of rats fed a protein-restricted diet during pregnancy suggests that reduced DNA methyltransferase-1 expression is involved in impaired DNA methylation and changes in histone modifications. Br J Nutr 2007;97(6):1064-1073

24. Burdge, GC. Et al. Dietary protein restriction of pregnant rats in the F0 generation induces altered methylation of hepatic gene promoters in the adult male offspring in the F1 and F2 generations. Br J Nutr 2007;97:435-439

Epigenetics of Diabetes

1. John Moffatt MD, Eight books on the causes, symptoms, and cure of acute and chronic diseases, translated from original Greek, London.pp204-209

2. Expert Committee on the Diagnosis and Classification of Diabetes Mellitus. Report of the expert committee on the diagnosis and classification of diabetes mellitus. Diabetes Care 2003;26:S5-S20

3. Mokdad, AH. Et al. Prevalence of obesity, diabetes, and obesity-related health risk factors, 2001. JAMA 2003:289:76-79

4. Brownlee, M., L.P. Aiello, M.E. Cooper, A.I. Vinik, R. Nesto, and A.J.M. Bolton. 2008. Diabetic Complications. In Williams Textbook of Endocrinology, 11th ed. Larsen, P.R., Kronenberg, H., Melmed, S., and Polonsky, K., editors. W.B. Saunders, Philadelphia. 1417–1501

5. Pirola, L. et al. Epigenetic phenomena linked to diabetic complications. Nature Reviews Endocrinology. 2010;6:665-675

6. El-Osta, A. et al. Transient high glucose causes persistent epigenetic changes and altered gene expression during subsequent normoglycemia. J Exp Med 2008;205(10):2409-2417

7. Holman, RR. Et al. 10 year follow-up of intensive glucose control in

type 2 diabetes. N Engl J Med 2008;359:1577-1589

8. Chalmers, J, Cooper, M. UKPDS and the legacy effect. N Engl J Med 2008;359:1618-1620

9. The Glycemic Index. The American Diabetes Association

10. Ludwig, DS. Dietary glycemic index and obesity. J Nutr 2000;130:280S-283S

11. Katan, MB. Et al. Beyond low fat diets. N Engl J Med 1997;337(8):563-566

12. Larson, DE. Et al. Dietary fat in relation to body fat and intraabdominal adipose tissue: a cross sectional analysis. Am J Clin Nutr 1996;64:677-684

13. Willett, WC. Is dietary fat a major determinant of body fat? Am J Clin Nutr 1998;67(Suppl):556S-562S

14. Daily dietary fat and total food-energy intakes—Third National health and nutrition examination survey, phase I, 1988-1991. Morbidity and Mortality Weekly Reports. 1994;43(7):116-117

15. Stephen AM, et al. Intake of carbohydrates and its components—international comparisons, trends over time, and effects of changing to low-fat diets. Am J Clin Nutr 1995;62:851S-867S

16. Mohindra, NA. et al. Eating patterns and overweight status in young adults: the Bogalusa Heart Study. Int J Food Sci Nutr 2009;60(suppl 3):14-25

17. Popkin, BM. Et al. Dietary changes in older Americans, 1977-1987. Am J Clin Nutr 1992;55(4):823-830

18. Estrich, D. et al. Effects of co-ingestion of fat and protein upon carbohydrate-induced hyperglycemia. Diabetes 1967;16(4):232-237

19. Welch, IM et al. Duodenal and ileal lipid suppresses postprandial blood glucose and insulin responses in man: possible implications for the dietary management of diabetes mellitus. Clin Sci (London) 1987;72:209-216

20. Wolever, T, Bolognesi, C. Prediction of glucose and insulin responses of normal subjects after consuming mixed meals varying in energy, protein, fat, carbohydrate and glycemic index. J Nutr 1996;126:2807-2812

Epigenetics of Heart Disease

1. How your heart works. University of Montana www.montana.edu/craigs/How%20Your%20Heart%20Works.htm

2. Heart Disease Facts. CDC.GOV

3. Feero, WG. Et al. Genomics of cardiovascular disease. N Engl J Med 2011;365:2098-2109

4. Do, R. et al. The effect of chromosome 9p21variants on cardiovascular disease may be modified by dietary intake: evidence from case/control and a prospective study. PLoS Medicine 2011;8(10):e1001106

5. Hu, FB. Et al. Trends in the incidence of coronary heart disease and changes in diet and lifestyle in women. N Engl J Med 2000;343:530-537

6. Loucks, EB. Et al. Life-course socioeconomic position and incidence of coronary heart disease: The Framingham offspring study. Am J Epidemiol 2009;169:829-836

7. Tobi, EW. Et al. DNA methylation differences after exposure to prenatal famine are common and timing- and sex-specific. Human Mol Genetics 2009;18(21):4046-4053

8. Zaina, S. et al. Nutrition and aberrant DNA methylation patterns in atherosclerosis: more than just hyperhomocysteinemia? J Nutr 2005;135:5-8

9. Pons, D, Jukemia JW. Et al. Epigenetic histone acetylation modifiers in vascular remodeling- new targets for therapy in cardiovascular disease. Netherlands Heart Journal 2008;16(1):30-32

Epigenetics of Cancer

1. Feinberg, AP. Vogelstein, B. Hypomethylation distinguishes genes of some human cancers from their normal counterparts. Nature 1983;301:89-92

2. Brower, V. Unravelling the cancercode. Nature 2011;471:S12-S13

3. Tycko, B. Epigenetic silencing in cancer. J Clin Invest 2000;105(4):401-407

4. Sharma, S. et al. Epigenetics of cancer. Carcinogenesis 2010;31(1):27-36

5. Esteller, M. Epigenetics of cancer N Engl J Med 2008;358:1148-1159

References Chapter 2:

1. Top 500 industries in the United States, CNN.
http://money.cnn.com/magazines/fortune/fortune500/2009/performers/industries/fastgrowers

2. Pharmaceutical Industry Income.
http://www.reuters.com/article/2009/05/13/idUS140811+13-May-2009+BW20090513

3. Pharmaceutical Industry Income.
http://www.reportlinker.com/p0118600/US-Pharmaceutical-Industry-Report-2008-2009.html

4. Stevens VJ, Long Term Weight Loss and Changes in Blood Pressure: Results of the Trials of Hypertension Prevention, Phase II. Ann Int Med 2001;134:1-11

5. Pfeiffer, M. et al. Effects of short-term vitamin D (3) and calcium supplementation on blood pressure and parathyroid hormone levels in elderly women. J Clin Endocrinol Metab 2001;86(4):1633-1637

6. Bischoff-Ferrari HA. Et al. Oral supplementation with 25(OH)D3 versus vitamin D3: effects on 25(OH)D levels, lower extremity function, blood pressure, and markers of innate immunity. J Bone Mineral Res 2012;27(1):160-169

7. The agouti gene. Animalgenetics.us/agouti.htm

8. Dolinoy, D. The Agouti Mouse Model: an epigenetic biosensor for nutritional and environmental alterations on the fetal epigenome. Nutr Rev 2008;66(Suppl 1):S7-11.

Healthy Benefits of Specific Foods

Green Tea

1. Chako SM. Et al. Beneficial effects of green tea: a literature review. Chinese Med 2010;5:13

2. Suzuki, J. et al. Tea polyphenols regulate key mediators on inflammatory cardiovascular diseases. Med Inflamm 2009;Article ID494928

3. Crespy, V. Williamson, G. A review of the health effects of green tea catechins in In Vivo animal models. J Nutr 2004;134:3431S-3440S

4. Masuda, M. et al. Effects of epigallocatechin-3-gallate on growth, epidermal growth factor signaling pathways, gene expression, and chemosensitivity in human head and neck squamous cell carcinoma cell lines. Clin Cancer Res 2001;7:4220-4229

5. Khafif, A. et al. Quantitation of chemopreventive synergism between (-) epigallocatechin-3-gallate and curcumin in normal, premalignant and malignant human oral epithelial cells. Carcinogenesis. 1998;19(3):419-424

6. Fang MZ. Et al. Tea polyphenol –epigallocatechin-3-gallate inhibits DNA methyltransferase and reactivates methylation-silenced genes in cancer cell lines. Cancer Res 2003;63:7563-7570

7. Lee, WJ. Et al. Mechanisms for the inhibition of DNA methyltransferases by tea catechins and bioflavonoids. Mol Pharm 2005;68:1018-1030

8. Yuasa, Y. et al. DNA methylation status is inversely correlated with green tea intake and physical activity in gastric cancer patients. Int J Cancer 2009;124:2677-2682

9. Fang, MZ. Et al. Dietary polyphenols may affect DNA methylation. J Nutr 2007;223S-228S

10. Yang, CS. Et al. Tea and cancer prevention: molecular mechanisms and human relevance. Toxic Appl Pharmacol 2007;224(3):265-273

11. Tsao, AS. Et al. Phase II randomized, placebo-controlled trial of green tea extract in patients with high risk oral premalignant lesions. Cancer Prev Res 2009;2:931-941

12. Joshi, et al. Skeletal fluorosis due to excessive tea and toothpaste consumption. Osteoporosis Int. 2011;22(9):2557-2560

Grapes

1. This, P. et al. Historical origins and genetic diversity of wine grapes. Trends Genetics 2006;22(9):511-519

2. Opie LH, Lecour S. The red wine hypothesis: from concepts to protective signaling molecules. Eur Heart J. 2007;28:1683-1693

3. Ferrieres, J. The French paradox: lessons for other countries Heart 2004;90:107-111

4. Speakman JR, Mitchell SE. Caloric restriction. Mol Aspects Med 2011;32(3):159-221

5. Kaeberlein, M. et. al. Substrate specific activation of sirtuins by resveratrol. J Biol Chem 2005;280(17):17038-17045

6. Qin W. et al. Resveratrol induced DNA methylation in ER+ breast cancer. Proc Amer Assoc Cancer Res 2005;46:abstract 2750

7. Rimbaud S. et al. Resveratrol improves survival, hemodynamics and energetics in a rat model of hypertension leading to heart failure. PLoS ONE 2011;6(10):e26391

8. Labinsky, N. et al. Vascular dysfunction in aging: potential effects of resveratrol, an anti-inflammatory phytoestrogen. Curr Med Chem 2006;13(9):989-996

9. Pillai, JB. Et al. Activation of SIRT1, a class III histone deacetylase, contributes to fructose feeding-mediated induction of the α-myosin heavy chain expression. Am J Physiol Heart Circ Physiol 2008;294:H1388-H1397

10. Papoutsis, AJ. Et al. Resveratrol prevents epigenetic silencing of BRCA-1 by the aromatic hydrocarbon receptor in human breast cancer cells. J Nutr 2010;140:1607-1614

11. Kuwajerwala, N. et al. Resveratrol induces prostate cancer cell entry into S phase and inhibits DNA synthesis. Cancer Res 2002;62:2488-2492

12. Zhang, J. et al. Resveratrol inhibits insulin responses in a SIRT1-

independent pathway. Biochem J. 2006;397:527

13. Pfister, JA et al. Opposing effects of sirtuins on neuronal survival: SIRT1-mediated neuroprotection is independent of its deacetylase activity. PLoS ONE 2008;3(12):e4090

14. Zhang, J et al. The type III histone deacetylase SIRT1 is essential for maintenance of T cell tolerance in mice. J Clin Invest 2009;119(10):3048-3058

15. Kruszewski,M. Szumiel L, Sirtuins (histone deaceytlases III) in the cellular response to DNA damage-facts and hypothesis. DNA Repair (Amst) 2005;4(11):1306-1313.

16. Dai Y, Faller, DV. Transcription regulation by class III histone deacetylases (HDACs)-Sirtuins. Trans Oncogenomics 2008;3:53-65

Flaxseed:

1. Flaxseed, Medline Plus. www.nlm.nih.gov/medlineplus/druginfo/natural/991.htm

2. Flaxseed, American Institute for Cancer Research. www.aicr.org/foods-that-fight-cancer/flaxseed.html

3. Flaxseed, the Natural Medicines Comprehensive Database www.naturaldatabase.therapeuticresearch.com

4. Leitzmann, MF et al. Dietary intake of n-3 and n-6 fatty acids and the risk of prostate cancer. Am J Clin Nutr 2004;80:204-216

5. Demark-Wahnefried, W et al. Flaxseed supplementation (not dietary fat restriction) reduces prostate cancer proliferation rates in men presurgery. Cancer Epidemiol Biomarkers Prev 2008;17:3577-3587

6. Tham, D et al. Potential health benefits of dietary phytoestrogens: a review of the clinical, epidemiological, and mechanistic evidence. J Clin Endocrinol Metab. 1998;83:2223-2235

7. Chen, JC. Et al. Flaxseed alone or in combination with tamoxifen inhibits MCF-7 breast tumor growth in ovariectomized athymic mice

with high circulating levels of estrogen. Exp Biol Med 2007;232:1071-1080

8. Lindahl G. et al. Tamoxifen, flaxseed, and the lignan enterolactone increases stroma and cancer cell derived IL-1Ra and decrease tumor angiogenesis in estrogen dependent breast cancer. Cancer Res 2011;71:51-60

9. Jungeström, MB et al. Flaxseed and its lignans inhibit estradiol-induced growth, angiogenesis, and secretion of vascular endothelial growth factor in human breast cancer xenografts in vivo. Clin Cancer Res 2007;13:1061-1067

10. Prasad K. Flaxseed and cardiovascular health. J Cardiovasc Pharmacol 2009;54(5):369-377

11. Bloedon, LT. et al. Flaxseed and cardiovascular risk factors: results from a double-blind, randomized, controlled clinical trial. J Am Coll Clin Nutr 2008;27(1):65-74

12. Aukema H. Effects of flaxseed on renal disease. Manitoba Agriculture, Food and Rural Initiatives. www.gov.mb.ca/agriculture/research/ardi/projects/01-515.html

Green Leafy Vegetables

1. Green Leafy Vegetables. Department of Agriculture, www.usda.gov

2. Nierenberg C. Leafy greens-ranked and rated. www.webmd.com/diet/healthy-kitchen-11/leafy-greens-rated

3. Pool-Zobel, BL. Et al. Mechanisms by which vegetable consumption reduces genetic damage in humans. Cancer Epidemiol Biomarkers Prev 1998;7:891-899

4. Doetsch PW. Et al. Nuclease SP: a novel enzyme from spinach that incises damaged duplex DNA preferentially at sites of adenine. Nucleic Acids Res 1988;16(14):6935-6952

5. Sacerdote, C. et al. Intake of fruits and vegetables and polymorphisms in DNA repair genes in bladder cancer. Mutagenesis 2007;22(4):281-285

6. Ribaya-Mercado, J. et al. Lutein and Zeanthin and their potential roles in disease prevention. J Am Coll Nutr 2004;23(6):567S-587S

7. Stidley, CA. et al. Multi-vitamins, folate, and green leafy vegetables protect against gene promoter methylation in the aerodigestive tract of smokers. Cancer Res 2010;70(2):568-574

Tomato

1. Tomatoes. Foods that Fight Cancer, American Institute for Cancer Research www.aicr.org

2. Carotenoids: alpha carotene, beta carotene, beta-cryptoxanthin, lycopene, lutein, zeanthin. Micronutrient Information Center. Linus Pauling Institute, Oregon State University, lpi.osu.edu/infocenter/phytochemicals/carotenoids

3. Agarwal, S. et al. Tomato lycopene and its role in human health and chronic diseases. CMAJ 2000;163(6):739-744

4. Heber, D. Lu, Q. Overview of mechanisms of action of lycopene. Exper Biol Med 2002;227:920-923

5. Kelkel, M. et al. antioxidant and anti-proliferative properties of lycopene. Free Radic Res 2011;45(8):925-940

6. Bub, A. et al. Moderate intervention with carotenoid-rich vegetable products reduces lipid peroxidation in men. J Nutr 2000;130:2200-2206

7. Rao, AV, Agarwal, S. Role of antioxidant lycopene in cancer and heart disease. J Am Coll Nutr 2000;19(5):563-569

Cruciferous Vegetables

1. Cruciferous vegetables. Foods that Fight Cancer, American Institute for Cancer Research. www.aicr.org

2. Cruciferous vegetables. Micronutrient Information Center. Linus Pauling Institute, Oregon State University,

lpi.osu.edu/infocenter/foods/cruciferous

3. Tang, L. et al. Cruciferous vegetable intake is inversely associated with lung cancer in smokers: a case-controlled study. BMC Cancer 2010:10:162

4. Murray, S. et al. Effect of cruciferous vegetable consumption on heterocyclic aromatic amine metabolism in man. Carcinogenesis. 2001;22(9):1413-1420

5. Clarke, JD. Et al. Multi-targeted prevention of cancer by sulforaphane. Cancer Lett 2008;269(2):291-304

6. Ding, Y. et al. Sulforaphane inhibits 4-aminobiphenyl-induced DNA damage in bladder cells and tissues. Carcinogenesis. 2010;31(11):1999-2003

7. Gross-Steinmeyer, K. et al. Sulforaphane- and phenethyl isothiocyanate-induced inhibition of aflatoxin B1-mediated genotoxicity of human hepatocytes: role of GSTM1 genotype and CYP3A4 gene expression. Toxicol Sci 2010;116(2):422-432

8. Tsai, JT. Et al. Suppression of inflammatory mediators by cruciferous vegetable-derived indole-3-carbinol and phenethyl isothyocyanate in lipopolysaccharide-activated macrophages. Mediators Inflammation 2010;Article ID 293642

9. Xiao, D. et al. Phenethyl isothiocyanate inhibits oxidative phosphorylation to trigger reactive oxygen species-mediated death of human prostate cancer cells. J Biol Chem 2010;285(30):26558-26569

10. Wu, X. et al. Isothiocyanates induce oxidative stress and suppress the metastasis potential of human non-small cell lung cancer cells. BMC Cancer 2010;10:269

11. Jakubikova, J. et al. Anti-tumor activity and signaling events triggered by the isothiocyanates, sulforaphane and phenethyl isothiocyanate, in multiple myeloma. Haematologica 2011;96(8):1170-1179

12. Yanaka, A. et al. Dietary sulforaphane-rich broccoli sprouts reduce colonization and attenuates gastritis in Helicobacter pylori-infected

mice and humans. Cancer Prev Res 2009;2:353-360

Stem Cells

1. Stem Cell Primer. Stemcells.NIH.gov/info/

2. da Silva Meirelles, L. et al. Mesenchymal stem cells reside in virtually all post-natal organs and tissues.Journal of Cell Science 2006;119:2204-2213

3. Kang, KS. The secret lives of stem cells: Unraveling the molecular basis of stem cell aging. Cell Cycle 2011;10(24):4187

4. Lui, L, Rando TA. Manifestations and mechanisms of stem cell aging. J Cell Biol 2011;193(2):257-266

5. Mansilla, E. et al. Could metabolic syndrome, lipodystrophy, and aging be mesenchymas stem cell exhaustion syndromes? Stem Cells International Volume 2011, article ID 943216

6. Goldschmidt-Clermont, PJ. Et al. Inflammation, stem cells and atherosclerosis genetics. Curr Opin Mol Ther 2010;12(6):712-723

7. Betrami, AP et al. Stem cell senescence and regenerative paradigms. Clinical Pharmacology & Therapeutics 2012;91(1):21-29

8. Bachstetter AD. Et al. Spirulina promotes stem cell genesis and protects against LPS induced declines in neural stem cell proliferation. PLos ONE 2010;5(5):e10496

9. Shytle RD et al. Effects of blue green algae extracts on the proliferation of human adult stem cells in vitro: a preliminary study. Med Sci Monit 2010;16(1):1-5

10. Bickford PC et al. Nutraceuticals synergistically promote proliferation of human stem cells. Stem Cells Dev 2006;15(1):118-123

11. Shytle RD et al. Oxidative stress of neural, hematopoietic, and stem cells: protection by natural compounds. Rejuvenation Res 2007;10(2):173-178

12. Acosta S et al. NT-020, a natural therapeutic approach to optimize spatial memory performance and increase neural progenitor cell proliferation and decrease inflammation in the aged rat. Rejuvenation Res 2010;13(5):581-588

13. Kaneko Y. et al. Acute treatment with herbal extracts provides neuroprotective benefits in In Vitro and In Vivo stroke models, characterized by reduced ischemic death and maintenance of motor and neurologic functions. Cell Med 2010;1(3):137-142

14. Zhang XM, et al. Folate deficiency induces neural stem cell apoptosis by increasing homocysteine In Vitro. J Clin Biochem Nutr 2009;45:14-19

15. Liu, H et al. Folic acid supplementation stimulates notch signaling and cell proliferation in embryonic neural stem cells. J Clin Biochem Nutr 2010;47:174-180

16. Ichim TE et al. Circulating endothelial progenitor cells and erectile dysfunction: possibility of nutritional intervention? Panminerva Medica 2010;52(2):suppl 1, 75-80

17. Kondo, T et al. Smoking cessation rapidly increases circulating progenitor cells in peripheral blood in chronic smokers. Aterioscler Thromb Vasc Biol 2004;24(8):1442-1447

18. Erbs S. et al. Exercise training in patients with advanced chronic heart failure (NYHA IIIb) promotes restoration of peripheral vasomotor function, induction of endogenous regeneration, and improvement of left ventricular function. Circ Heart Fail 2010;3:486-494

19. Jensen GS. Et al. Mobilization of human CD 34+ CD 133 + and CD 34+ CD 133- stem cells in vivo by consumption of an extract from Aphanizomenon flos-aquae—related to modulation of CXCR4 expression by an L-selectin ligand? Cardiovasc Revasc Med 2007;8(3):189-202

20. Huang, PH. Et al. Intake of red wine increases the number and functional capacity of circulating endothelial progenitor cells by enhancing nitric oxide bioavailability. Arterioscler Thromb Vasc Biol 2010;30:869-877

21. Gorbunov N, et al. Regeneration of infarcted myocardium with resveratrol-modified cardiac stem cells. J Cell Mol Med 2012;16(1):174-184

21. Yasuhara, T et al. Dietary supplementation exerts neuroprotective effects in ischemic stroke model. Rejuvenation Res 2008;11(1):201-214

22. www.stemenhancefaq.com

23. www.stem-kine.com

IMMUNE SYSTEM

1. Schindler, L. et al. Understanding the immune system: Understanding cancer and related topics. National Cancer Institute Cancer.gov

2. Chandra RK. Nutrition and the immune system: an introduction. Am J Clin Nutr 1997;66:460S-463S

3. Müller, O. Krawinkel M. Malnutrition and health in developing countries. CMAJ 2005;173(3):279-286

4. Schaible, UE. Kaufmann SHE. Malnutrition and infection: Complex mechanisms and global impacts. PLoS Medicine 2007;4(5):806-812

5. Hendricks KM. et al. Malnutrition in hospitalized pediatric patients: Current prevalence. Arch Pediatr Adolesc Med 1995;149(10):1118-1122

6. Scheinfeld N. Protein Energy Malnutrion. http://emedicine.medscape.com/article/1104623-clinical

7. Micronutrient Information Center, Linus Pauling Institute, http://lpi.oregonstate.edu/infocenter/

8. Caulfield, LE et al. Stunting, wasting, and micronutrient deficiency disorders. Disease Control Priorities in Developing Countries, 2 Ed. Jamison DT, Breman JG, et. al, Editors Washington DC : World Bank 2006. Chapter 28, pp551-567

9. Lamm D. Riggs DR. Enhanced immunocompetance by garlic: Role in bladder cancer and other malignancies. J Nutr 2001;131:167S-1070S.

10. Ren Z. et al. White button mushroom enhances maturation of bone marrow-derived dendritic cells and their antigen presenting function in mice. J Nutr 2008;138:544-550

11. Lull C. et al. Antiinflammatory and immunomodulating properties of fungal metabolites. Mediators Inflammation 2005;2:63-80

12. Akramiene, D. et al. Effects of beta-glucans on the immune system. Medicina (Kaunas) 2007;43(8):597-606

13. Borchers AT. Et al. The immunobiology of mushrooms. Exp Biol Med 2008;233:259-276

14. Fish Oil. NIH, National Library of Medicine, Medline. http://www.nlm.nih.gov/medlineplus/druginfo/natural/993.html

15. Lovaza.com

16. Damsgaard CT. et al. Fish oil supplementation modulates immune function in healthy infants. J Nutr 2007;137:1031-1036

17. Hughes DA, Pinder AC. N-3 polyunsaturated fatty acids inhibit the antigen-presenting function of human monocytes. Am J Clin Nutr 2000;71(Suppl):357S-360S

18. McMurray DN et al. Effects of dietary n-3 fatty acids on T cell activation and T cell receptor-mediated signaling in a murine model. J Infect Dis 2000;182(suppl 1):S103-S107

19. Kim H. Glutamine as an immunonutrient. Yonsei Med J 2011;52(6):892-897

20. Glutamine. WebMD.com, vitamins and supplements

21. Xiao-Yu L. Immunomodulating Chinese herbal medicines. Mem Inst Oswaldo Curz 1991;86 Suppl II:159-164

22. Sun, Y. et al. Immune restoration and/or augmentation of local graft versus host reaction by traditional Chinese medicinal herbs. Cancer 1983;52(1):70-73

23. Chu, DT et al. Immunotherapy with Chinese medicinal herbs. I. Immune restoration of local xenograft graft-versus-host reaction in

cancer patients by fractionated Astragalus membranaceous in vitro. J Clin Lab Immunol 1988;25(3):119-123

24. Chu, DT et al. Immunotherapy with Chinese medicinal herbs. II. Reversal of cyclophosphamide-induced immune suppression by administration of fractionated Astragalus membranaceous in vivo. J Clin Lab Immunol 1988;25(3):125-129

25. Oral Probiotics: an introduction. National Center for Complementary and Alternative Medicine.
http://nccam.nih.gov/health/probiotics/introduction/htm

26. Evrard B. et al. Dose-dependent immunomodulation of human dendritic cells by the probiotic Lactobacillus rhamnosus Lcr35. PLoS ONE 2011;6(4):e18735

27. Shida K. et al. Flexible cytokine production by macrophages and T cells in response to probiotic bacteria. Gut Microbes 2011;2(2):109-114

28. Galdeano CM. et al. Impact of probiotic fermented milk in the gut ecosystem and in the systemic immunity using a non-severe protein-energy-malnutrition model in mice. BMC Gastroenterology 2011;11:64

29. Lata, J. et al. Probiotics in hepatology. World J Gastroenterol 2011;17(24):2890-2896

30. Thurnham DJ. Micronutrients and immune function: some recent developments. J Clin Pathol 1997;50:887-891

31. High KP. Micronutrient supplementation and immune function in the elderly. Clin Infectious Dis 1999;28:717-722

32. Prasad AS. Zinc: mechanisms of host defense. J Nutr 2007;137:1345-1349

33. Prasad AS. Zinc in human health: Effect of zinc on immune cells. Mol Med 2008;14(5-6):353-357

34. Prasad AS. et al. Zinc supplementation decreases incidence of infections in the elderly: effect of zinc on generation of cytokines and oxidative stress. Am J Clin Nutr 2007;85:837-844

35. Schwalfenberg, GK. A review of the critical role of vitamin D in the

functioning of the immune system and the clinical implications of vitamin D deficiency. Mol Nutr Food Res 2011;55:96-108

36. Hewison, M. Vitamin D and the immune system: new perspectives on an old theme. Endoc Metab Clin North Am 2010;39(2):365-379

References Chapter 3:

1. Ulijaszek, SJ. Et al. Human dietary change (and discussion). Phil Trans Roy Soc Lond. B 1991;334:271-279

2. Dr. Scott Olson ND, Sugarettes, Wellbright LLC. 1998

3. What do Americans eat? U.S. Agriculture Fact Book 1998, Chapter 1a

4. USDA Fact Book 2000

5. Americans consume too much salt. Centers for Disease Control and Prevention. http://www.cdc.gov/Features/dsSodium/

6. Nine in 10 Americans eat too much salt: CDC Reuters.com 6-24-2010

7. David Kessler MD, Rodale MD, The End of Overeating. Rodale Books. 2009

8. Kuczmarski, RJ.et al. Increasing prevalence of overweight among US adults. JAMA 1994;272(3):205-211

9. Flegal, KM. et al. Prevalence of trends in obesity among US adults 1999-2008. JAMA 2010;303(3):235-241

10. The truth about fad diets. WebMD.com
http://www.webmd.com/diet/guide/the-truth-about-fad-diets

Paleolithic/Hunter-Gatherer Diet

1. O'keefe, JH. Cordain, L. Cardiovascular disease resulting from a diet and lifestyle at odds with our paleolithic genome: How to become a 21st Century Hunterer-Gatherer. Mayo Clin Proc 2004;79:101-108

2. Eaton, SB, Konner, M. Paleolithic nutrition. N Engl J Med. 1985;312(5):283-289

3. Milton, K. The critical role played by animal food source foods in human (Homo) evolution. J Nutr 2003;3886S-3892S

4. Cordain, L. et al. Plant-animal subsistence ratios and macronutrient energy estimations in worldwide hunter-gatherer diets. Am J Clin Nutr 2000;71:682-692

5. Cordain, L. et al. The paradoxical nature of hunter-gatherer diets: meat-based, yet non-atherogenic. Eur J Clin Nutr 2002;56(Suppl 1):S42-S52

6. Osterdahl, M. et al. Effects of short-term intervention with a paleolithic diet in healthy volunteers. Eur J Clin Nutr 2008;62(5):682-685

7. Frassetto, LA et al. Metabolic and physiologic improvements from consuming a paleolithic, hunter-gatherer type diet. Eur J Clin Nutr 2009;63(8):947-955

8. O'Dea, K. Marked improvement in carbohydrate and lipid metabolism in diabetic Australian aborigines after temporary reversion to traditional lifestyle. Diabetes 1984;33(6):596-603

9. Lindeberg, S. et al. A paleolithic diet improves glucose tolerance more than a Mediterranean-like diet in individuals with ischaemic heart disease. Diabetologia 2007;50:1795-1807

10. Jönsson, T. et al. Beneficial effects of Paleolithic diet on cardiovascular risk factors in type 2 diabetes: a randomized cross-over pilot study. Cardiovasc Diabetology 2009;8:35

Low Carbohydrate/Atkins-like diet

1. Dr. Atkins Diet Revolution, Dr. Robert Atkins, Bantam Publishers 1972

2. Dr. Atkins New Diet Revolution, Dr. Robert Atkins, Harper Publishers 2002

3. The Atkins Diet, Mayoclinic
http://www.mayoclinic.com/health/atkins-diet/MY08

4. Duda, MK. Et al. Low carbohydrate/high fat diet attenuates pressure overload induced ventricular remodeling and dysfunction. J Card Fail 2008;14(4):327-335

5. Brinkworth, GD. Et al. Effects of a low carbohydrate weight loss diet on exercise capacity and tolerance in obese subjects. Obesity 2009;17:1916-1923

6. Frisch, S. et al. A randomized controlled trial on the efficacy of carbohydrate-reduced or fat-reduced diets in patients attending a telemedically guided weight loss program. Cardiovasc Diabetology 2009;8:36

7. Bradley, U. et al. Low-fat versus low-carbohydrate weight reduction diets. Diabetes 2009;58:2741-2748

8. Phillips, SA. Et al. Benefit of low-fat over low-carbohydrate diet on endothelial health in obesity. Hypertension 2008;51(2):376-382

9. Brinkworth, GD. Et al. Long-term effects of a very-low-carbohydrate weight loss diet compared with an iso-caloric low-fat diet after 12 Mo. Am J Clin Nutr 2009;90:23-32

10. Hernandez, TL. Et al. Lack of suppression of circulating free fatty acids and hypercholesterolemia during weight loss on a high-fat low-carbohydrate diet. Am J Clin Nutr 2010;91:578-585

11. Comparative effects of 3 popular diets on lipids, endothelial function, and C-reactive protein during weight maintenance. J Am Diet Assoc 2009;109(4):717-717

12. Rankin, JW, Turpyn, AD. Low-carbohydrate high-fat diet increases C-reactive protein during weight loss. 2007;26(2):163-169

13. Al-Sarraj, T et al. Carbohydrate restriction, as a first-line dietary intervention, effectively reduces biomarkers of metabolic syndrome in Emirati adults. J Nutr 2009;139:1667-1676

14. Foster, GD. Et al. Weight and metabolic outcomes after 2 years on a low-carbohydrate versus low-fat diet. Ann Intern Med 2010;153(3):147-157

15. Kodama, S. et al. Influence of fat and carbohydrate proportions on the metabolic profile in patients with type 2 diabetes: a meta-analysis. Diabetes Care 2009;32:959-965

Dash Diet

1. Blumenthal, JA. Et al. Effects of the DASH diet alone or in combination with exercise and weight loss on blood pressure and cardiovascular biomarkers in men and women with high blood pressure: The ENCORE Study. Arch Intern Med 2010;170(2):126-135

2. Hypertension Guidelines, National Institutes of Health. http://www.nhlbi.nih.gov/guidelines/hypertension/jnc7full.pdf

3. Sacks, FM et al. Effects on blood pressure of reduced dietary sodium and the dietary approaches to stop hypertension (DASH) diet. N Engl J Med 2001;344:3-10

4. The DASH diet. Dashdiet.org

5. Shenoy, SF. Et al. Weight loss in individuals with metabolic syndrome given DASH diet counseling when provided a low sodium vegetable juice: a randomized controlled trial. Nutr J 2010;9:8

6. Fung, TT. Et al. Adherence to a DASH-style diet and risk of coronary heart disease and stroke in women. Arch Intern Med 2008;168(7):713-720

7. Levitan, EB. Et al. Consistency with the DASH diet and incidence of heart failure. Arch Intern Med 2009;169(9):851-857

8. Taylor, EN. DASH-style diet associates with reduced risk for kidney stones. J Am Soc Nephrol 2009;20:2253-2259

9. Fung, TT. Et al. Low-carbohydrate diets, dietary approaches to stop hypertension-style diets, and the risk of postmenopausal breast cancer. Am J Epidemiol 2011;174(6):652-660

Mediterranean Style Diet

1. Trichopoulou, A. et al. Adherence to a Mediterranean diet and survival in a Greek population. N Engl J Med 2003;348:2599-2608

2. Hu, FB. The Mediterranean diet and mortality- olive oil and beyond. N Engl J Med 2003; 348:2595-2596

3. Mozafarrian, D, Wu, JH. Omega-3 fatty acids and cardiovascular disease: effects on risk factors, molecular pathways, and clinical events. J Am Coll Cardiol 2011;58(20):2047-2067

4. Bullo, M. et al. Mediterranean diet and oxidation: nuts and olive oil as important sources of fat and antioxidants. Curr Top Med Chem 2011;11(14):1797-1810

5. Perona, JS. Et al. The role of virgin olive oil components in the modulation of endothelial function. J Nutr Biochem 2006;17:429-445

6. Estruch, R. et al. Effects of Mediterranean-style diet on cardiovascular risk factors: a randomized trial. Ann Intern Med 2006;145:1-11

7. Esposito, K. et al. Effects of Mediterranean-style diet on the need for anti-hyperglycemic drug therapy in patients with newly diagnosed type 2 diabetes. Ann Intern Med 2009;151:306-314

8. de Lorgeril, E. et al. Mediterranean alpha-linoleic acid-rich diet in secondary prevention of coronary heart disease. Lancet 1994;343(8911):1454-1459

9. Kavouras, SA. Et al. Physical activity and adherence to Mediterranean diet increase total antioxidant capacity: the ATTICA study. Cardiol Res Practice 2011: article ID 248626

10. Esposito, K. et al. Long-term effect of Mediterranean-style diet and calorie restriction on biomarkers of longevity and oxidative stress in overweight men. Cardiol Res Practice 2011:article ID 293916

11. Paoli, A. et al. Effect of ketogenic Mediterranean diet with phytoextracts and low carbohydrates/high-protein meals on weight, cardiovascular risk factors, body composition and diet compliance in Italian council employees. Nutrition Journal 2011;10:112

12. Sofi, F. et al. Accruing evidence on benefits of adherence to the Mediterranean diet on health: an updated systemic review and meta-analysis. Am J Clin Nutr 2010;92:1189-1196

13. Wu, AH. Et al. Dietary patterns and breast cancer risk in Asian American women. Am J Clin Nutr 2009;89:1145-1154

14. Fung, TT. Et al. Diet quality is associated with the risk of estrogen receptor-negative breast cancer in postmenopausal women. J Nutr 2006;136:466-472

15. Trichopoulou, A. et al. Conformity to traditional Mediterranean diet and breast cancer risk in the Greek EPIC (European Prospective Investigation into Cancer and Nutrition) cohort. Am J Clin Nutr 2010;92:620-625

16. Buckland, G. et al. Adherence to a Mediterranean diet and the risk of gastric adenocarcinoma within the European Prospective Investigation into Cancer and Nutrition (EPIC) cohort study. Am J Clin Nutr 2010;91:381-390

17. Ferris-Tortajada, J et al. Dietetic factors associated with prostate cancer. Protective effects of Mediterranean diet. Actas Urol Esp 2011, Sep 27, EPUB ahead of print

18. Shai, I. et al. Weight loss with a low-carbohydrate, Mediterranean, or low fat diet. N Engl J Med. 2008;359:229-241

19. Sacks, FM. Et al. Comparisons of weight-loss diets with different compositions of fat, protein, and carbohydrates. N Engl J Med 2009;360:859-873

Vegetarian/Vegan Diets

1. Key, TJ, et al. Health effects of vegetarian and vegan diets. Proc Nutr Soc 2006;65:35-41

2. Craig, WJ. Health effects of vegan diets. Am J Clin Nutr 2009;89(Suppl):1627S-1633S

3. Hunt, IF. Et al. Bone mineral content in postmenopausal women: comparison of omnivores and vegetarians. Am J Clin Nutr 1989;50:517-523

4. Ho-Pham, LT. et al. Effect of vegetarian diets on bone mineral density: a Bayesian meta-analysis. Am J Clin Nutr 2009;90:943-950

5. Lantham-New, SA. Is "vegetarianism" a serious risk factor for

osteoporotic fracture? Am J Clin Nutr 2009;90:910-911

6. Thorpe, DL. Et al. Effects of meat consumption and vegetarian diet on risk of wrist fracture over 25 years in a cohort of peri- and postmenopausal women. Public Health Nutr 2008;11(6):564-572

7. Fraser, GE. Vegetarian diets: what do we know of their effects on common chronic diseases? Am J Clin Nutr 2009;89(Suppl):1607S-1612S

8. Craig, WJ. Nutrition concerns and health effects of vegetarian diets. Nutr Clin Pract 2010;25:613-620

9. Sabaté, J. Nut consumption, vegetarian diets, ischemic heart disease risk, and all-cause mortality: evidence from epidemiologic studies. Am J Clin Nutr 1999;70(Suppl):500S-503S

10. Fernandes-Dourado, K. et al. Relation between dietary and circulating lipids in lacto-ovo vegetarians. Nutr Hosp 2011;26(5):959-964

11. Yang, SY. Et al. Relationship of carotid intima-media thickness and duration of vegetarian diet in Chinese male vegetarians. 2011;8:63

12. Crowe, FL. Et al. Diet and risk of diverticular disease in Oxford cohort of European Prospective Investigation into Cancer and Nutrition (EPIC): prospective study of British vegetarians and non-vegetarians. BMJ 2011;343:d4131

13. Tonstad, S. et al. Type of vegetarian diet, body weight, and prevalence of type 2 diabetes. Diabetes Care 2009;32:791-796

14. Barnard, ND. Et al. A low-fat vegan diet and a conventional diabetes diet in the treatment of type 2 diabetes: a randomized, controlled, 74 week trial. Am J Clin Nutr 2009;89(Suppl):1588S-1596S

15. Jenkins, DJA. Et al. The effect of a plant-based low-carbohydrate ("eco-Atkins") diet on body weight and blood lipid concentrations in hyperlipidemic subjects. Arch Intern Med 2009;169(11):1046-1054

16. Sabaté, J, Wien, M. Vegetarian diets and childhood obesity prevention. Am J Clin Nutr 2010;91(suppl):1525S-1529S

17. Singh, PN. Et al. Does low meat consumption increase life expectancy in humans? Am J Clin Nutr 2003;78(suppl):526S-532S

18. Chang-Claude, J. et al. Lifestyle determinants and mortality in German vegetarians and health-conscious persons: results of a 21-year follow-up. Cancer Epidemiol Biomarkers Prev 2005;14:963-968

19. Key, TJ. Et al. Mortality in British vegetarians: review and preliminary results from EPIC-Oxford. Am J Clin Nutr 2003;78(Suppl):533S-538S

Supplements

1. Morbidity and Mortality Weekly Reports, Surveillance data 2009, CDC.gov

2. Reduce your risk of cancer. http://www.aicr.org/reduce-your-cancer-risk/recommendations-for-cancer-prevention/recommendations_04_plant_based.html

3. 5-a-day may not be enough. http://www.webmd.com/heart-disease/news/20110118/5-a-day-not-enough-fruits-vegetables

4. Use of dietary supplements on the rise. http://www.webmd.com/diet/news/20110413/use-of-dietary-supplements-on-the-rise?src=RSS_PUBLIC

5. AICR press release Feb 11, 2008

6. http://www.heart.org/HEARTORG/GettingHealthy/NutritionCenter/Vitamin-and-Mineral-Supplements_UCM_306033_Article.jsp

7. Thomson, MJ. Et al. Antioxidant treatment for heart failure: friend or foe? Q J Med 2009;102:305-310

8. Bleys, J. et al. Vitamin-mineral supplementation and the progression of atherosclerosis: a meta-analysis of randomized controlled trials. Am J Clin Nutr 2006;84:880-887

9. Cuerda, C. et al. Antioxidants and diabetes mellitus: review of the evidence. Nutr Hosp 2011;26(1):68-78

10. Neuhouser, ML. et al. Dietary supplement use and prostate cancer risk in the Carotene and Retinol Efficacy Trial. Cancer Epidemiol

Biomarkers Prev 2009;18(8):2202-2206

11. Lippman, SM. Et al. Effect of selenium and vitamin E on risk of prostate cancer and other cancers: The Selenium and Vitamin E Cancer Prevention Trial (SELECT). JAMA 2009;301(1):39-51

12. Fritz, H. et al. Vitamin A and retinoid derivatives for lung cancer: a systematic review and meta-analysis. PLoS ONE 2011;6(6):e21107

13. Omenn, GS. Et al. Effects of combination of betacarotene and vitamin A on lung cancer and cardiovascular disease. N Engl J Med 1996;334:1150-1155

14. Hennekens, CH. Et al. Lack of effect of long-term supplementation with beta-carotene on the incidence of malignant neoplasms and cardiovascular disease. N Engl J Med. 1996;334(18):1145-1149

15. Soni, MG. et al. Safety of vitamins and minerals: controversies and perspective. Toxicological Sci 2010;118(2):348-355

16. Bjelakovic, G. et al. Mortality in randomized trials of antioxidant supplements for primary and secondary prevention. JAMA 2007;297:842-857

17. Fairfield, KM, Fletcher, RH. Vitamins for chronic disease prevention. JAMA 2002;287:3116-3126

Whole Food Supplements

1. Arendt, BM. Et al. Plasma antioxidant capacity of HIV-seropositive and healthy subjects during long-term ingestion of fruit juices or a fruit-vegetable-concentrate containing antioxidant polyphenols. Eur J Clin Nutr 2001;55:786-792

2. Otsuka, T. et al. Suppressive effects of fruit-juice concentrate of Prunus mume Sieb. et Zucc. (Japanese apricot, Ume) on Helicobactor pylori-induced glandular stomach lesions in Mongolian gerbils. Asian Pacific J Cancer Prev 2005;6:337-341

3. Dai, Q. et al. Fruit and vegetable juices and Alzheimer's disease: the Kame project. Am J Med 2006;119(9):751-759

4. Jensen, GS. Et al. Pain reduction and improvement in range of motion after daily consumption of an Acai (Euterpe oleracea Mart.) pulp-fortified polyphenolic-rich fruit and berry juice blend. J Med Food 2011;14(7/8):702-711

5. Esfahani, A. et al. Health effects of mixed fruit and vegetable concentrates: a systematic review of the clinical interventions. J Am Coll Nutr 2011;30(5):285-294

6. Ruxton, CH. Et al. Can pure fruit and vegetable juices protect against cancer and cardiovascular disease too? A review of the evidence. Int J Food Sci Nutr 2006;57(3-4):249-272

7. De Spirt, S. et al. An encapsulated fruit and vegetable juice concentrate increases skin microcirculation in healthy women. Skin Pharmacol Physiol 2012;25:2-8

8. Nantz, MP. Et al. Immunity and antioxidant capacity in humans is enhanced by consumption of a dried, encapsulated fruit and vegetable juice concentrate. J Nutr 2006;136:2606-2610

9. Chapple, ILC. Et al. Adjunctive daily supplementation with encapsulated fruit, vegetable and berry juice powder concentrates and clinical periodontal outcomes: a double-blind RCT. J Clin Periodontol 2012;39:62-72

10. Jin, Y. et al. Systemic inflammatory load in humans is suppressed by consumption of two formulations of dried, encapsulated juice concentrate. Mol Nutr Food Res 2010;54(10):1506-1514

11. Novembrino, C. et al. Effects of encapsulated fruit and vegetable juice powder concentrates on oxidative status in heavy smokers. J Am Coll Nutr 2011;30(1):49-56

12. Samman, S. et al. A mixed fruit and vegetable concentrate increases plasma antioxidant vitamins and folate and lowers plasma homocysteine in men. J Nutr 2003;133:2188-2193

13. Kiefer, I. et al. Supplementation with mixed fruit and vegetable juice concentrates increased serum antioxidants and folate in healthy adults. Kiefer, I. et al. 2004;23(3):205-211

14. Lamprecht, M. et al. Several indicators of oxidative stress, immunity, and illness improved in trained men consuming an encapsulated juice powder concentrate for 28 weeks. J Nutr 2007;137:2737-2741

15. Roll, S. et al. Reduction of common cold symptoms by encapsulated juice powder concentrate of fruits and vegetables: a randomized, double-blind, placebo-controlled trial. Br J Nutr 2011;105:118-122

16. Zhang, J. The effect of fruit and vegetable powder mix on hypertensive subjects: a pilot study. J Chiropractic Med 2009;8:101-106

References Chapter 4:

Micronutrients

1. Office of Dietary Supplements, National Institutes of Health

2. Modern Nutrition in Health and Disease; Lipincott, Williams, and Wilkins 10 Ed.

References:

Nancy Gibbs. The Magic of the Family Meal, TIME 2006;June 4

ABOUT THE AUTHOR

Dr. Bob Avery currently practices Hematology and Oncology in Alabama. He completed medical school at St. Louis University and trained in Internal Medicine and Hematology/Oncology in the U.S. Army. It was during his tour in Germany that he became interested in complementary medicine and nutrition. He is married and has five wonderful children.

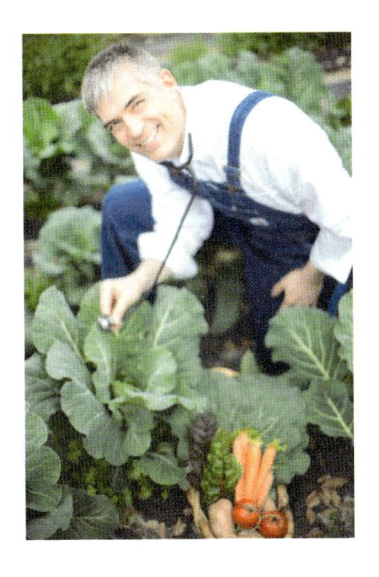

Contact: AskDrAvery@citrinesun.com
Youtube: DrBobCitrineSun
Blog: www.Citrinesun.com

Made in the USA
Lexington, KY
31 January 2013